THE NEW SCHOOL HEALTH HANDBOOK

A Ready Reference for School Nurses and Educators

Jerry Newton, M.D.

Director, Health Services
San Antonio Independent School District
San Antonio, Texas

Clinical Professor, Pediatrics
University of Texas Health Science Center
of San Antonio

Illustrations by John Martini, MSMI

Prentice Hall
Englewood Cliffs, New Jersey

Prentice-Hall International (UK) Limited, *London*
Prentice-Hall of Australia Pty. Limited, *Sydney*
Prentice-Hall Canada, Inc., *Toronto*
Prentice-Hall Hispanoamericana, S.A., *Mexico*
Prentice-Hall of India Private Limited, *New Delhi*
Prentice-Hall of Japan, Inc., *Tokyo*
Simon & Schuster Asia Pte. Ltd., *Singapore*
Editora Prentice-Hall do Brasil, Ltda., *Rio de Janeiro*

10 9 8 7 6 5 4 3 2 1

Library of Congress Cataloging-in-Publication Data

Newton, Jerry, 1920–
   The new school health handbook: a ready reference for school
nurses and educators/Jerry Newton; illustrations by John Martini.
   p.   cm.
   Rev. ed. of: School health handbook. c1984.
   Includes index.
   ISBN 0-13-615923-0
   1. Pediatrics—Handbooks, manuals, etc.   2. School children—
Diseases—Handbooks, manuals, etc.   3. Child health services—
Handbooks, manuals, etc.   I. Newton, Jerry, 1920–   School health
handbook.   II. Title.
   [DNLM: 1. Pediatrics—handbooks.   2. School Health Services—
handbooks.   WS 39 N564s]
RJ48.N48   1989
618.92'0008837—dc19
DNLM/DLC
for Library of Congress   89–3675
                                                                 CIP

ISBN 0-13-615923-0

PRENTICE HALL
BUSINESS & PROFESSIONAL DIVISION
A division of Simon & Schuster
Englewood Cliffs, New Jersey 07632

Printed in the United States of America

ABOUT THE AUTHOR

Jerry Newton, a pediatrician with a wide variety of experiences, conducted a busy private practice in San Antonio, Texas, for twenty-three years. This was followed by three years of bouncing around in a jeep as a Peace Corps physician in Paraguay, where he not only was the personal physician to seventy-five Peace Corps volunteers, but also the medical supervisor for the Peace Corps Public Health Program in Paraguay.

On returning to the United States, he became the full-time medical director of the San Antonio Independent School District and has served in that position for over fifteen years. Many school districts have medical consultants, but in only a few is the physician an active member of the superintendent's staff. Moving through the corridors of ninety schools and constant contact with school nurses, principals, and teachers have given him an unusual insight into the special medical problems of school children and the need for better health education.

He has consistently applied his efforts to improve the quality of health care offered to students. To increase the effectiveness and expand the services provided by school nurses, he developed an active school nurse practitioner program, which has resulted in many new and innovative school health programs and clinics dealing with learning disabilities and behavior problems.

Dr. Newton is Clinical Professor of Pediatrics at the University of Texas Medical School in San Antonio and has been active in school health committees of his local and state medical associations as well as the American School Health Association and the American Academy of Pediatrics. He is the author of *School Health Handbook: A Ready Reference for School Nurses and Educators* (Prentice–Hall, 1984) and *Complete Book of Forms for the School Health Professional* (Prentice–Hall, 1987). He is the editor of School Health Alert, the only monthly newsletter that deals solely with comprehensive school health: services, education, and environment, and which is read by over 3000 school nurses and educators.

ABOUT THIS NEW EDITION

Now more than ever before, school health services have become indispensable in large urban school districts as well as in many smaller urban, suburban, and rural schools. This new revised and expanded edition of the *School Health Handbook* deals with all the revolutionary changes in school health service.

The New School Health Handbook is written primarily for the licensed professional school nurse. Medical jargon has been eliminated as much as possible; when used, it is explained so that nonmedical personnel can use the book, too.

In school districts with budgetary constraints and a shortage of nurses, vocational or practical nurses step in to fill the need. When no nurse is on campus, the principal or secretary must substitute in her absence, having to make health decisions that will possibly need to be defended later.

School administrators can also use this book to assist in formulating policy and as a guide for making recommendations to school board members.

Expanded Role of the Professional School Nurse

The professional school nurse is the obvious person in the school system to act as interpreter between the educational and medical communities and to offer suggestions for the management of each individual child, as well as for health service programs for the school district as a whole.

● *The school nurse must practice independently.* The school nurse is expected to know etiology, epidemiology, differential diagnosis, proper treatment, and other aspects of managing health problems in children. School nurses, through their professional organizations, have developed training programs designed to refresh their basic skills and adapt them to carry on these functions in a school setting. This is quite different from a hospital in which support personnel, equipment, and physical design are all geared to health care rather than education. The revisions of and additions to *The New School Health*

Handbook will enable the school nurse, with her background and experience, to interpret and carry out the doctor's orders in a manner most appropriate to the student in school. Also, more independent decisions, based on scientific knowledge, will be possible.

● *New sections address the profound changes required to implement the mandates of PL 94-142 (education for all handicapped children).* School nurses are familiar with the problems of acutely ill children—their fevers, runny noses, coughs, and stomach aches. However, the child with moderate and severe developmental disabilities, who would never have been in school five or ten years ago, now is routinely placed in a classroom at the youngest legal age, usually three years. The numbers of seriously and profoundly disabled children in school have become so large that even the smallest school districts are feeling the impact of this law. The passage of PL 99-457 in 1986 will soon extend services to children under three years of age as well. Skilled, professional nursing care is essential during school hours—administration of medicine, tube feeding through mouth and gastrostomy, catheterization, tracheostomy care and suctioning, changing of ostomy bags, and other hospital procedures are now routinely done in school.

● *The nurse's interaction with therapists.* Children with severe mental, emotional, and physical disabilities (and various combinations thereof) are utilizing a larger percentage of the school budget. The demand for health-related services such as occupational therapy, physical therapy, and speech therapy has exploded. School systems are hard put to find this type of skilled employee in sufficient numbers and at reasonable cost to satisfy the demands of parents and physicians. Schools need help to understand which types of disabilities will benefit from the various therapies advocated, when the therapy should be initiated, and when it may be stopped.

● *Additional problems, previously not school concerns.* With the leap in numbers of teenage unmarried mothers, working mothers, and single-parent families, schools are assuming a larger parenting role, especially in three areas: (1) day care centers for babies of students, (2) before- and after-school child care, and (3) health services. When the child gets sick at school, there may not be anyone at home to receive the child. The increase in the adolescent and preadolescent pregnancy rate in the U.S., now the largest in the developed world, challenges the schools to "do something about it." One response, in addition to more health and sex education, has been the school-based clinic. At the time of this book's writing, there are over 100 such programs in the U.S.

● *New chapters on contagious diseases on campus.* The spread of AIDS and the admission of children with AIDS to school has opened a whole new area of school health concerns. Related to this are diseases such as cytomegalovirus, hepatitis B, rubella, and herpes simplex, which if contracted while pregnant may be passed to the unborn baby. Young, mentally retarded children have a higher incidence of these diseases, are capable of spreading the virus, and are now attending school. Classroom teachers, students, and aides are concerned that they may be exposed, especially if they are pregnant.

The Revised Edition

The twenty sections of *The New School Health Handbook* address all of these changes and concerns and serve as a resource and reference for school health professionals, directors of special education, and school administrators.

Jerry Newton, M.D.

CONTENTS

Section 3

DISEASES OF THE EARS, NOSE, AND THROAT ● 39

Section 4

EYE PROBLEMS ● 49

Section 5

DISEASES OF THE LUNGS ● 62

Section 6

DISEASES OF THE HEART • 75

Section 7

DISEASES OF THE BRAIN • 85

Section 8

DISEASES WITH SPECIAL SCHOOL RELEVANCE • 103

Section 9

CHRONIC TRANSMISSIBLE NEONATAL INFECTIONS ● 131

Section 10

BITES AND STINGS ● 141

Section 11

DIABETES • 149

Section 12

COMMON CHILDHOOD RASHES • 159

Section 13

SCHOOL-RELATED EMOTIONAL/SOCIAL PROBLEMS • 167

Section 14

BEHAVIOR DISORDERS ● 193

Section 15

PSYCHOACTIVE MEDICATIONS COMMONLY USED
FOR CHILDREN • 219

Section 16

DISORDERS OF LEARNING • 231

Section 17

HEALTH SCREENING PROGRAMS • 257

Section 18

INJURIES ● 279

Section 19

CLINIC EMERGENCIES • 310

Section 20

SEVERE PHYSICAL DISABILITIES • 337

ADMINISTRATIVE ASPECTS OF SCHOOL HEALTH

School Nurses
- Historical Background
- Relationship to School Personnel
- School Nurse Functions

Physician Consultants
- Communicating With Physicians
- Information the Doctor Needs from School
- Choosing a Doctor

Medical Excuses
- Types
- Role of the School Nurse
- Standing Orders and Nursing/Medical Protocols

SCHOOL NURSES

Historical Background

For many years school health services have been provided by municipal health departments through the employment of city or county public health nurses. In many cities and counties, this arrangment still exists and adequately serves school health needs. In some communities, however, as the demand for other public health nursing services has grown, school health services provided by municipalities have declined. In the past twenty to thirty years, many school districts have created their own departments of health services, with school nurses, supervisors, and consulting or full-time medical doctors. The school nursing profession has developed high standards, programs providing a variety of services have become fairly well standardized throughout the states, and the past fifteen years has seen a large increase in health services to the handicapped.

Relationship to School Personnel

Though it is important for school nurses to know how schools, principals, counselors, and teachers function, the school nurse's expertise is not, nor should it be, in education. Traditional school in-service programming rarely applies to the school nurse. School nurses must be given opportunities for professional renewal if they are to be of value to the school system. There are national and state organizations of school nurses, and each school nurse should be encouraged to join and to attend meetings.

Health services in most public schools are administratively separated from health education. Health service is considered a support service staffed largely by school nurses, whereas health education is part of the general education curriculum. This type of administrative arrangement tends to separate the school nurse from the formal educational process. To effectively utilize their expertise, forward-looking health educators often use school nurses as resource people when teaching about drug use and abuse, infectious diseases, wonder drugs such as penicillin, menstruation, hygiene, nutrition, and other appropriate subjects. In addition, there is, among school nurses, a movement to improve their qualifications. Many school districts require their nurses to have baccalaureate degrees; school nurse practitioners and nurse specialists are more numerous.

The future holds great promise for an expansion of the school nurse's role. Most disabled school children require the services of both health and education specialists. In the United States, the entire field of education, which in the past has limited itself primarily to teaching, is providing ever increasing care for disabled children. In order to provide such health care, there will be an increasing demand for the services of school nurses.

Because the school nurse is the person on campus who has a medical background, she can most effectively become the liaison between the educational and medical communities. If she stays currently informed and is willing to assume the role of "school health guardian," she can be alert for dangers as they are reported: storage and preparation of food, food additives, sugar substitutes; toxic art supplies; tampons, playground equipment and precautions, sources of lead and other toxins; etc.

Also, the nurse should be current on information regarding health screening procedures (scoliosis, vision, etc.) and immunizations. It was because I became aware of the need for schools to have this information that I now publish the *School Health Alert Newsletter* which summarizes current health information for the school nurse.

The following are a few of the many scientifically reliable publications to which every school should subscribe for its nurse:

- *FDA Consumer,* a monthly magazine, uses lay language and is scientifically reliable. Write to:
  Superintendent of Documents
  Government Printing Office
  Washington, D.C. 20402
- *MMWR (Morbidity and Mortality Weekly Reports)* is published weekly by the Centers for Disease Control. It uses technical language, provides up-to-the-minute information, and is highly reliable. For regular delivery, write to:
  Massachusetts Medical Society
  CSPO Box 9120
  Waltham, MA 02254-9120
  (880) 843-6356
  First Class $40; Third Class $26
  annually

For more rapid delivery of *MMWR,* write to:

> Superintendent of Documents
> Government Printing Office
> Washington, D.C. 20402
> (202) 783-3238
> First Class $69 annually

- *PDR (Physicians' Desk Reference)* offers information concerning pharmaceutical products. It is issued annually and contains technical language. Write to:

> Medical Economics Company Inc.
> 680 Kinderkamack Road
> Oradell, NJ 07649

- *Drug Evaluations,* issued annually, gives information concerning pharmaceutical products. Write to:

> American Medical Association
> 535 N. Dearborn Street
> Chicago, IL 60610

School Nurse Functions

In addition to giving first aid in the school clinic, school nurses also perform many screening tests such as vision, hearing, height, weight, pulse, and blood pressure, on appropriate groups of children. Other functions include visits to homes and neighborhood clinics in order to follow the course of children with chronic illness. Immunizations are very important in childhood. In some school districts nurses actually give immunizations, while in others they ensure that all children have had the immunizations required by law and refer parents to where they may be obtained: public health clinics, private doctors, and neighborhood health centers. Emerging specialized functions performed by nurses with varying degrees of advanced training are:

1. Evaluation of the medical aspects of children with learning and behavior problems. Since school nurses have both medical expertise and educational exposure they are able to evaluate the medical history, the socioeconomic status, the physical condition, and the relationship of all these factors to the child's learning style and behavioral pattern.

2. Special physical screening programs, such as complete physical examinations on school entry and scoliosis (spinal curvature) screening in early adolescence.

3. Special vision screening procedures in addition to the standard visual acuity testing. Examples are tests for eye muscle imbalance and excessive hyperopia.

4. Liaison between educational and medical personnel, especially with regard to special education placement and development of the individual educational plan.

5. Medical evaluation procedures that help assess developmental levels of young children, since standard educational pencil-and-paper psychometric testing is inaccurate and difficult in very young children (ages two through four years).

6. Work with occupational and physical therapists in the care of disabled children.

PHYSICIAN CONSULTANTS

Communicating with Physicians

When a child has a clear-cut medical illness for which he or she is receiving adequate medical attention through the family doctor, school personnel are usually informed of the progress and nature of the disease, and there is no need for additional direct communication. However, a student may have a medical condition for which the school nurse may feel the need to talk to the doctor directly. There are two categories of such conditions:

1. Some chronic low-grade illnesses permit children to continue school attendance, but various symptoms (poor appetite, failure to play) may cause the teacher to suspect they are not doing as well as they should.

2. Some learning and behavior problems are sufficiently serious to require medical intervention. In cases of this nature, school nurses often need to talk to the doctor to give input that will supplement that of the parents. In addition, the nurse is often seeking advice that will help in the child's management and education.

Because of laws governing medical confidentiality, a doctor will require written parental consent to disclose information to the school. Therefore, the nurse must talk to the parent first and obtain permission to contact the doctor. Most parents are glad to cooperate. After obtaining the necessary permission form, the nurse should mail it to the doctor. The nurse should then call the doctor's secretary, make sure the release form has arrived, and explain the nature of the call. If the above procedure is followed, the school nurse will usually receive cooperation from the doctor.

As all experienced school nurses know, things do not always go smoothly. Some of the obstacles are created by:

- An uncooperative or poorly informed parent.
- The absence of a reliable and regular source of medical care.
- Doctors who cannot be reached by phone (often employed by large city, county or military hospitals, or health care businesses).
- An uncooperative doctor. Some doctors have very little or no familiarity with the administrative and professional operation of a school.

Some medical schools and postgraduate medical training programs are beginning to incorporate some public school health experience into their programs in the hope that physicians will become better acquainted with school personnel and practices and will be more understanding of school problems.

Information the Doctor Needs from School

Some doctors are baffled when asked to see children who have been referred for learning or behavior disorders. They cannot understand why school authorities would refer a "well" child to them, and they often diagnose the child as free of disease. The child will return to school with a note containing the diagnosis "normal." Doctors who are knowledgeable about school diagnostic procedures and management methods can be most helpful. Copies of psychometric test results, achievement tests, teacher evaluation of the child's behavior are essential. Also, a written two-or-three-day chronological account of the child's actions over a period of an hour or two each day is necessary. This account must be strictly objective and report only the child's actions, not the observer's opinions or inferences. It should describe actions in two or three locations, such as in class, in the cafeteria, in line, or on the playground. The doctor will also need to know what the school expects from the medical evaluation—what specific deficits or defects are medically related and whether the doctor can help ameliorate the problem.

Sometimes the problem is simple, clear-cut, and easy to remedy. For example, a six year old child with classical attentional deficit disorder, obvious hyperactivity and no apparent emotional problems should respond well to medication. Such a case presents little problem in communication between school and doctor. However, a ten year old who won't do homework, has almost illegible handwriting, talks back to the teacher, and is one or two grades below the class level, presents a much more difficult problem and requires a great deal of bilateral cooperation between school and doctor. Carefully selective neurological evaluation may reveal poor muscular control, inability to get things in their proper sequence, or poor spatial arrangement ability. There may be undiscovered emotional problems that are manifested as school failure.

Choosing a Doctor

Pediatricians are most likely to be knowledgeable about and interested in school problems. A pediatrician who has special interest or extra training in behavioral or developmental pediatrics will be most helpful. The Society for Behavioral Pediatrics, 241 E. Gravers Lane, Philadelphia, PA, (212) 305-9862 can provide the name of a nearby member. Pediatric neurologists and child psychiatrists also deal with this category of disorder, but usually they see cases on referral from pediatricians or family practitioners.

If you chose a doctor by letting your fingers walk through the yellow pages, you may improve your odds slightly by considering that recently trained doctors are more apt to be knowledgeable about learning disorders and school-related problems. Passing specialty board exams (American Board of Pediatric, American Academy of Family Practice, etc.) and having a medical school appointment increase the chances that the doctor will have had some training regarding medical-educational problems. You can call the office of the local county medical society to ascertain these factors.

Beyond this, you must judge the doctor's personal qualities: returning phone calls, being available when needed, showing a genuine interest in the child, and making real efforts to help by providing sufficient time when necessary to discuss complicated problems.

If the student is receiving dependent's care at a military base, enrolled in a large health maintenance organization (HMO), or a large city/county hospital, it is usually best to deal with a patient-care coordinator or one of the nurses in charge of the clinic the child is attending.

MEDICAL EXCUSES

Types

The medical excuses that children or their parents bring to school from a doctor's office vary from a hastily scrawled note on a prescription slip to a formal letter. They can be categorized as follows:

1. *Excuses for acute or chronic illnesses for specific periods of time.* These periods may be long or short, but in either case usually cause no school administrative problems. The school nurse knows (or can find out) that the child is legitimately ill and can suggest steps to be taken to ensure the child's continuing education.

2. *Excuses from gym class.* Some of the more common reasons doctors furnish are:

- Excuses for the whole school year for unspecified reasons
- Excuses for obesity
- Excuses for diseases with an emotional component, such as asthma
- Excuses for children who are said to catch cold easily in cold or cool weather

As a rule, doctors do not realize that physical education is a required high school course in most states. Doctors acknowledge the benefit of regular exercise but they know that missing an occasional gym classes will not have a deleterious effect on a child's health. Occasionally there are emotional or psychological factors that doctor and patient feel are better kept private.

There are irregularities and injustices on both sides of this issue. Physicians in private practice have seen many children who had a perfectly legitimate reason for being excused from gym classes, who in

one way or another received prejudicial treatment for bringing medical excuses. On the other hand, school nurses have seen many children
bring hastily scrawled notes from doctors asking for a whole year's
excuse for reasons that were clearly not valid.

3. *Excuses to permit change of school.* Most school districts require a
student to attend the school within the geographic boundaries of the
attendance zone. Usually, a medical or psychological reason contained
in a note from a doctor will be considered sufficient grounds for a
transfer to another school. Nevertheless, many of these transfer
requests are arguable. Sometimes a child wants to go to another school
to be with a friend. Sometimes the other school is near a relative where
the child can go after school until the parents get home from work.
The child may not want to be bused out of his or her neighborhood or
into a strange one. Again, in these cases most doctors don't realize the
constraints and pressures school authorities work under. Often a
principal has denied a transfer request to one student and then has to
justify granting one to another, especially if everyone in the neighborhood knows that the second student is not sick in any way but has a
compliant physician who simply writes excuses to satisfy a demanding
parent. Some excuses are justified, and some are not. It is necessary to
investigate each case individually; the school nurse can help the
principal in this investigation.

Role of the School Nurse

There are no easy general answers that apply to every case, but
there are certain helpful guidelines.

1. Any note that excuses a child from physical education for the
whole year on vague grounds should be closely questioned.

2. Ease of catching cold, mild asthma, and controlled epilepsy are
not legitimate reasons for avoiding all gym classes. They *are* reasons
for adapting the exercises so they are safe and not too strenuous.

3. Emotional factors are important; physical deformity and obesity must be considered in this category. If a student has a legitimate
reason for not disrobing or wearing gym clothes, and the doctor is
sincerely trying to help the student, then the nurse and the gym
teacher should try their best to cooperate by communicating with the

doctor, discussing both sides of the situation, and arriving at a satisfactory solution.

4. It is not necessary for a child to "suit up" to participate in gym class. Failure to change clothes should not lower a child's grade if the reasons are legitimate. A student can participate in an adaptive physical education program in regular school clothes. Many middle school and high school principals condone this practice.

Standing Orders and Nursing/Medical Protocols

Since almost all states have laws that prohibit nurses from making a medical diagnosis and prescribing treatment, there are differing feelings among school nurses concerning the legality of diagnosing and/or identifying obvious medical conditions or illnesses. For example, school nurses do not hesitate to identify (or diagnose) head lice; some feel competent to identify impetigo, scabies, or chicken pox, but most will not diagnose diseases such as hepatitis or scarlet fever.

In the early 1970s for differing reasons, school nurses began to expand their scope of activities. Since then, the identification in school of conditions such as scabies, lice, impetigo, strep throat, and other minor illnesses has increasingly been done by the school nurse.

The school nurse practitioner movement began in the early 1970s and received impetus a few years later from a $5–$6 million Robert Wood Johnson grant. Also, the school-based clinic movement, which began in Dallas, Texas and St. Paul, Minnesota in 1967, has expanded rapidly, especially since 1984–85, due to the large increase in teen pregnancy. At this time there are over 100 such clinics in the U.S. In these school clinics, a school nurse practitioner, under a physician's supervision, diagnoses and treats certain minor illnesses commonly seen in schools. The nurse follows protocols or a set of standing orders dated and signed by the physician supervisor. Medical and nursing practice laws permit these special arrangements in some states.

Some school districts with part-time, full-time, or consulting physicians have developed their own sets of standing orders, not only to help the school nurse to provide more efficient health services, but also to give the nurse better legal protection. In this process, each school district, with input from nurses, doctors, and school administrators, develops its unique protocols and set of standing orders. (See Figures 1–1 and 1–2.)

Figure 1–1. Sample—Lengthy and Detailed Protocol (This type of description is often used when nurses work in relatively isolated areas and more independent decisions must be made.)

IMPETIGO

Definition

Superficial infection of the skin manifested by vesicular or pustular lesions that rapidly become crusted.

Etiology

Caused by certain strains of streptococci, staphylococcus, or by a combination of both.

Epidemiology

Can occur at any age; both sexes and all races equally vulnerable. It is often associated with poor hygiene and is contagious. Infection is spread by contact with material from skin lesions.

Clinical Manifestations

Onset usually sudden; may be prolonged with new lesions developing over several months if child is not treated.

Lesions tend to occur at site of previous injury (scratch) and at mucocutaneous junctions (corner of lip, nasal folds); common on fingers.

Red macule-vesicle-pustule-crust lesions vary in size. Multiple sites can appear readily and diffusely. Lesions are superficial because bacteria invade upper skin layers.

May have pruritus, regional adenopathy, low-grade fever.

Diagnosis

Culture of material from pustule on blood agar, rarely necessary. Lesions as described above.

Treatment

1. Antibiotic therapy for 10 days (only necessary for severe cases)
   a. Pen-Vee-K 50–100 mg/kg/day

   b. Erythromycin 20–40 mg/kg/day q.i.d. × 10 days if allergic to penicillin and no history of erythromycin sensitivity

2. Wet compresses to crusts with careful removal t.i.d. by parent
3. Bacitracin ointment
4. Urinalysis 2–4 weeks after prescription ends or as need arises
5. Heart exam 2–4 weeks after prescription
6. Throat culture of patient and family if impetigo recurs

Prognosis

Excellent

Complications

1. Ecthyma—more serious form of impetigo with deeper invasion of streptococcus into dermis—results from neglect and poor general physical resistance.
2. Cellulitis.
3. Acute glomerular nephritis. Efficacy of penicillin therapy in preventing acute glomerular nephritis is questionable but strongly advocated at present.

Education

1. Explain carefully to parents dosage of antibiotic and importance of compliance (A.G.N.).
2. Stress importance of child's fingernails being kept short and clean.
3. Discourage scratching.
4. All involved in child's care should wash hands carefully.
5. Child's towel and wash cloth must be isolated.
6. Classmates, relatives, siblings should be observed carefully for suspicious lesions.
7. Report any change in condition (antibiotic intolerance, lesions, urinary complaints, etc.).
8. Child may attend school if under treatment for 24 hours.

Read and approved by:

Date:

Adapted from "Protocols for Nurse Practitioner," Robert Wood Johnson School Health Project, Newburgh, New York

Figure 1–2. Sample—Concise Protocol

IMPETIGO

Physical findings

1. Primary lesion is a vesicle that rapidly becomes pustular.
2. Honey-colored, loosely adherent crusts.
3. Occasionally liquid or crusted pustules.
4. Most frequently found on fingers and face but may be anywhere on body.
5. Itching.
6. Contagious on direct or secondary contact.
7. Deeper lesions with thick adherent crusts called ecthyma.

Treatment

1. Bacteria live under the crusts.
2. Gently wash with soap or septisol, and remove as much of crust as possible.
3. Apply direct pressure until bleeding stops after removal of crust.
4. Apply bacitracin ointment.
5. Cover with dressing or adhesive bandage.
6. Keep fingernails short.
7. Refer moderate to severe cases to physician.
8. May attend school if under treatment.

Follow-up

1. See in clinic daily until healing process well under way.
2. Watch for cellulitis.
3. Watch for furunculosis.
4. Watch for systemic illness with fever.

Read and approved by:

Date:

Listed below are conditions frequently described in school health services protocols and standing orders:

1. Abrasions
2. Acne
3. Anaphylaxis
4. Asthma
5. Blunt injury, abdomen
6. Blunt injury, chest
7. Boils
8. Burns
9. Cellulitis and lymphangitis
10. Common colds vs. allergic rhinitis
11. Conjunctivitis
12. Contact dermatitis
13. Dog bite and human bite
14. Eczema
15. Enuresis, encopresis
16. Foreign bodies
17. Heal trauma
18. Herpes simplex
19. Hives, urticaria, laryngeal edema
20. Impetigo
21. Lacerations
22. Nosebleed
23. Ringworm, tinea
24. Scabies
25. Seizures, epilepsy
26. Sprain, ankle or knee
27. Sty

SECTION 2

DISEASES OF THE SKIN

Head Lice
- Nature of the Condition
- Symptoms
- Diagnosis
- Treatment
  —Medications
  —Mechanical Methods
- Action by School Personnel

Scabies
- Nature of the Condition
- Symptoms and Diagnosis
- Complications
- Treatment and Role of the School Nurse

Ringworm
- Four Classes of Ringworm
  —Tinea Capitis
  —Tinea Pedis
  —Tinea Curis
  —Tinea Corporis
- Treatment in General

Impetigo
- Nature of the Condition
- Treatment

Paronychia or "Felon"
- Nature of the Condition
- Symptoms
- Treatment and Role of the School Nurse

Boils (Furuncles)
- Nature of the Condition
- Symptoms
- Treatment
- Role of the School Nurse

Acne
- Nature of the Condition
- Symptoms
- Emotional Problems
- Treatment
- School Relevance and Role of the School Nurse

Herpes Simplex
- Nature of the Condition
- Symptoms
- Modes of Transmission
- Treatment
- Prevention
- School Relevance and Role of the School Nurse

HEAD LICE

Nature of the Condition

Because of a vast resurgence in the past twenty to twenty-five years, head lice infestation is probably the largest and most exasperating problem in schools today.

The adult head louse (pediculosis capitis) is about 1/16 inch long and gray. It crawls fairly fast. It cannot jump like a flea.

The adult female louse lays eggs (nits) at the base of the hair shaft right next to the scalp. The egg is then covered with a tiny bit of gelatinous material that hardens into a semi-opaque, tiny pearly, whitish mass that is stuck tight to the hair shaft. In about seven to ten days, the egg matures and hatches into a louse that lives by sucking blood from the scalp. Without a human host, it can live one to three days without a blood meal. Each adult lives about one to three weeks, and a female can lay eggs several times before it dies of old age.

The biggest problem with lice is *reinfestation,* especially when siblings share the same bed. The nits resist treatment and hatch live lice. Products used on the hair vary in effectiveness; those with a smaller kill ratio need to be left on longer. Some kill both adult lice and nits.

Symptoms

In severe cases, one usually sees a child with dirty hair which is matted and unkempt. Scratching is prominent. Closer inspection reveals nits and live, crawling lice.

In mild cases, the hair may appear to be clean and combed if one merely views the child from a distance. Suspicion may be aroused by scratching, and on close inspection nits can be seen.

If lice infestation is neglected, a child's head can look pretty bad. The excessive scratching causes a secondary infection from germs normally present on the scalp, such as staphylococcus. These infected areas of matted hair will require frequent washing and applications of antibiotic ointment. Occasionally some of the hair must be cut away.

Lymph nodes in the neck will often be swollen. Scratching fingers may also transfer the infection from the scalp to other parts of the child's body, even affecting (rarely) internal organs such as the liver and spleen.

Diagnosis

Severe cases are obvious by simply looking at the child's head. Mild cases will require a closer inspection. If an instrument like a pencil is used to separate the hair, care must be taken not to convey the message that the child is too dirty to touch; the child has no control over the problem. A fastidious teacher may be required to act cooler than he or she feels. The examination should be done unobtrusively and privately. When possible, school staff should refer the child to the school nurse for diagnostic confirmation—the nurse is, alas, a lice expert.

Teachers may have an aversion to handling a head that houses "crawlers," but there is no reason to fear catching them. Lice can't jump on you, and nits are stuck to the hair. Physicians and other health workers have handled hundreds of infested children without catching lice.

There are several ways to tell the difference between nits and dandruff. A louse usually lays the egg on the hair close to the scalp; a scale of dandruff may be an inch or two away. However, in warm climates, the nits may be deposited farther from the scalp. A nit is stuck to the hair shaft and will not shake off as dandruff will. However, an old nit that has hatched will leave behind a shell that will shake loose. If there is doubt, recheck the child's head in a day or two, or pluck the suspected hair and look at it under a good light.

Treatment

Medications

All medicines used are applied to the hair; none are taken internally. They fall into two categories: 1% lindane lotion and pyrethrins.

Lindane. The common trade-mark brand is "Kwell." The generic is also available. The PDR recommends lindane or Kwell *lotion* be used for scabies, allowing it to remain on the body eight to twelve hours. The *shampoo* is recommended for lice and that it remain on the head for only four minutes. This is illogical; both the lotion and shampoo contain 1% lindane—the only difference is the carrier. It is my opinion that the four-minute contact time recommended for Kwell shampoo is the reason for the reportedly high failure rate. There have been sporadic anecdotal reports from California and England that head lice are developing a resistance to lindane. This has not yet been confirmed. (*CA Morbidity*, 1/24/86, 4/17/87)

Pyrethrins. "Rid" and "Nix" are well known. Nix is a pyrethr*oid*, a synthetic product, said to be more stable and, at this writing, thought to be most effective. It still requires a prescription, is not generic, and is expensive—about $13–$16 for a 2 oz. bottle.

No medicine, prescription or nonprescription, should be used unless it has been recommended by a physician, school nurse, or other health expert. For example, if a child has many sores and Kwell is applied, it may be absorbed into the bloodstream and cause serious complications.

After one treatment with an effective medication, the child should be able to attend school the next day.

Mechanical Methods

Simply washing the hair with soap and water every day will completely eliminate head lice in ten to fourteen days. Another method is to use a good-grade hair dryer. Lice are killed (or stunned) at about 120 to 140 degrees Fahrenheit. Hot air from a hair blower will cause the hatched crawlers to fall off.

Many products are sold to spray clothes, furniture, and other household items. Save your money. Those sprays are rarely helpful. *Never* use a spray on a child.

The only sure way to eliminate all nits is to soften them with vinegar or similar substance and comb them out with a fine-tooth comb. In a child with thick long hair, this is difficult or impossible. They will fall off in a few days anyway.

Action by School Personnel

Should the child, once lice are discovered, be sent home immediately? In some schools one-fourth of the class would be sent home if a diligent search were made. It has been advocated that children with even a few nits and no adult live lice should be sent home. In my opinion this is unrealistic and unnecessary. Some cases obviously need immediate isolation, but in the average public school, I would not routinely send every case home.

Public health laws in almost all states require exclusion of children with many contagious diseases. Schools, however, recognize degrees of contagiousness and are usually allowed discretion in complying with these statutes. Just as with mild colds, sore throats, ringworm, or impetigo—all of which are contagious diseases—if one were to search out and send home all diagnosed cases, too many children would be involved. It's much more practical to send home a note at the end of the school day and save the heavy ammunition (parent conference with the principal or three-day suspensions) for those rare, severe cases in which the parents are completely uncooperative or obstructive. In cases of this nature, the total school management becomes more of an administrative than a medical problem. Not only the principal, but often upper-level school administrators, as well as the PTA, could be involved.

SCABIES

Nature of the Condition

Scabies, the original "seven-year itch," is caused by a tiny mite, too small to be seen by the naked eye. In past years it was largely seen in military barracks, orphanages, and other institutions. It was uncommon between the late 1930s and 1960s, but is now frequent throughout the United States and is prevalent in many schools. Because it was a rarity for some thirty years, many physicians did not encounter it in their private practice and now may fail to recognize it.

Since the mites live underneath the skin, contagion takes rather prolonged contact, such as children sleeping in the same bed or two children wrestling. A nurse or teacher need never be concerned about touching a child who has scabies—one simply will not get scabies in this manner. All that is required for safety is washing the hands after touching a child with scabies (or lice). Scabies (and lice) are an occupational nuisance rather than a hazard of the teaching profession. School nurses and teachers need to associate and play with children as part of their professional life. On the rare occasions when a teacher does get scabies, it is very easy to cure and should not occasion undue alarm.

Symptoms and Diagnosis

The adult mite burrows beneath the skin of humans and animals. (In dogs and cats, it causes mange.) The mite makes a tiny white bump that itches intensely, particularly at night. As a result of scratching, a scab ½ to 1 millimeter long appears on the skin. The scab tends to be linear rather than round, and this aids in the diagnosis. Another characteristic of scabies is its location on the body. It is commonly found on the backs of the hands, the webs between the fingers, the inner side of the wrist and forearms, and the chest and abdomen. If there are no sores on any of these places, scabies can probably be ruled out. It can also be found on the upper arms and legs, and the neck. It is practically never on the face, on the small of the back between the shoulder blades, on the palms of the hands, or on the soles of the feet. It will often be found on more than one member of the family.

Complications

One of the major complications of scabies is impetigo, an infection of the outer layer of the skin where germs (staphylococcus or streptococcus) normally live. Impetigo is the inevitable result of continued scratching. Once established, it can spread over a large area of the skin surface, become quite severe, and cause more of a problem than the scabies itself. In order to cure this type of scabies, one must first cure the impetigo.

Treatment and Role of the School Nurse

Scabies is easy to cure. Treatment consists of applying one of several different kinds of lotions or ointments, the most effective being lindane lotion, the same one that is used for head lice. The standard method is to apply the lotion from the chin line down to the toes, covering the entire body. The instructions are always outlined in the package insert or can be obtained from the family doctor or school nurse. It is left on for six to eight hours, and then the child is given a bath. The average infestation of scabies will be cured by one application. Some children with severe infestation require two treatments, which should be at least seven days apart. Babies should be clothed so they do not lick their skin. Bed linens and all of the child's clothing should be washed through an ordinary wash cycle in the washing machine. This will eliminate any live scabies, mites, or eggs that might be present. Other methods of treatment, such as benzyl benzoate or sulfur, are effective but rarely used nowadays.

A child with scabies presents no immediate emergency and need not be sent home. By the time the disease is discovered, it has already existed (and has been contagious) for several days or weeks. At the end of the school day, send a note to the parent stating that the child has a contagious skin condition and should not be sent back to school until treated. Remember the sensibilities of the child. Spare him or her any social discomfort by your reaction, and keep your discovery confidential from the other students.

RINGWORM

Four Classes of Ringworm

Ringworm (*tinea*) is a fungus infection of the skin, which is most commonly found in four areas of the body:

1. Scalp—*tinea capitis*
2. Feet—*tinea pedis* (athlete's foot)
3. Genital area—*tinea cruris* (jock itch)
4. Trunk, face, and limbs—*tinea corporis*

Though all four are caused by similar fungi, the appearance and treatment are different depending on the location.

Tinea Capitis

Nature of the Condition

The infected scalp typically has small patches of baldness (1–3 inches in diameter) that may well be unnoticed under long hair. Boys and girls are equally susceptible, but almost never after puberty. Since the infection affects the hair shaft itself, close inspection reveals tiny, broken-off hairs about ¹⁄₁₆ to ⅛ inch long.

Treatment

The treatment for tinea capitis is always oral medication. Topical ointments will cure ringworm of the body and feet but not of the scalp. The generic name of the oral medicine is griseofulvin, and in many cases it only takes a few days of treatment to render the child noncontagious, even though it takes four to ten weeks of treatment for a complete cure.

Recent studies indicate that the type of fungus which commonly causes tenia capitis is changing; in some cases it may take 2-3 weeks of griseofulvin therapy to render a child noncontagious. This will be a serious problem, because a hair or scalp culture for fungus takes one to two weeks to grow, meaning that if exclusion procedures are strictly enforced, the child could miss three to five weeks of school.

Differentiating Alopecia Areata

Tinea capitis is often confused with another condition called *alopecia areata,* which also causes round bald spots. In the latter case, the bald spots are absolutely smooth with no broken hairs; the hair falls out by the roots. The differentiation is important because alopecia areata is completely noncontagious, whereas tinea capitis is one of the most contagious of all diseases and can spread through a school rapidly if not controlled. Any suspicious case should be referred to the principal and the school nurse so the child can be sent to the doctor immediately and not allowed back in school until diagnosed and under treatment.

Role of the School Nurse

School nurses will need to deal with individual doctors and develop strategies such as having the student wear a head covering until the fungus is no longer active. In addition, she should inspect the child's head periodically to make sure improvement continues. Many children fail to take long-term medications regularly.

Tinea Pedis

Athlete's foot is much more common in boys than in girls. It responds easily to appropriate lotions or ointments, but unfortunately, it keeps coming back in certain susceptible individuals. Many men never completely get rid of it.

Gym teachers are most aware of this condition and usually prepare a solution for the children to step into before going to the showers. While this does no harm, it doesn't really help. Schools that still follow this practice should have the solution cultured periodically to make sure the fungus isn't actually growing in it. Children with obvious sores on their feet should be sent to the school nurse or personal physician for treatment.

Tinea Curis

This type of ringworm, found in the folds and creases of the body, especially the groin area, is often called jock itch. It is more common in obese individuals, both boys and girls. It is usually quite uncomfortable, itches intensely, and is worse in the summer.

Jock itch is usually caused by various fungi. It is easy to cure, but, like athlete's foot, it often comes back. Cleanliness and certain lotions will cure it very quickly.

Tinea Corporis

Ringworm of the body is common. It appears on the arms, chest, and abdomen, and more rarely on the face. It starts as a tiny red spot, which slowly grows in a circular fashion, clearing in the center as it enlarges. The edges remain reddish and scaly. No scabs, pus, or crusts are formed as in impetigo. Most children have a single lesion, but on occasion, a child will develop more.

Children often develop small, round, whitish depigmented areas on their cheeks and upper arms. This is definitely not ringworm and is not contagious. Its cause is unknown, but it waxes and wanes without treatment and is completely harmless. If one looks carefully, it is easy to see that the edges of the whitish circular area look the same as the center, thus distinguishing it from ringworm.

Treatment in General

Ringworm of the body, feet, and groin can be treated easily with medicines like tolnaftate (Tinactin), chlortrimazole (Lotrimin), and related compounds. They are not greasy and do not sting the skin or smell bad. Iodine and merthiolate can also be used, but they may sting. The first treatment renders children noncontagious so they can stay in school during treatment until the sores are gone. As stated before, if the scalp is involved, it is necessary to take medicine internally, and it takes two to five days or more to become noncontagious.

IMPETIGO

Nature of the Condition

Impetigo is a bacterial infection, usually caused by staphylococcus germs, which invades the upper layer of the skin. Probable causes are lowering of body resistance (questionable), hot humid weather (more likely), and excess scratching because of lice, insect bites, or scabies (very common). It is more common in children who wash and bathe less frequently.

The most characteristic features of impetigo are the honey-colored and red scabs that cover all or part of each sore. These crusts are easy to pick off or rub off, but usually some bleeding occurs when this is done. The sores may be single and isolated, about ½ inch in diameter, or several may coalesce and form a larger, irregularly shaped sore. Sores are common where children always scratch themselves—on the face, on the fingers, and around the nose. Usually, the palms and soles will be spared.

Since many children have impetigo and it is usually only contagious on direct contact, if there are only a few sores they can be treated and covered with an adhesive bandage, and the child can remain in school. A child with many exposed, visible lesions may have to be sent home.

Treatment

Treatment of impetigo usually requires two steps. First, one must rub or pick off the scab. The germs live under it, and this is where the medicine must be applied. This step hurts a little bit but is necessary. One should soften the scab by soaking and washing the sores with soap and water, then rub hard with gauze or a wash rag. Let the child apply pressure until the small amount of bleeding stops (three to five minutes). One removal is usually sufficient, but if the scab builds up again it may be necessary to repeat the process. Many minor cases can be cured by this treatment alone.

The second step is to apply a little antibacterial ointment (bacitracin is the one most commonly used) and cover with an adhesive bandage if desired. This should be done two to three times a day until the condition is cured. It usually takes only a few days. Other simple antiseptics like merthiolate will also cure small single sores.

It is important to treat impetigo because the sores can continue to spread. In rare cases the germs may find their way into internal organs and cause abscesses (boils) to form in such vital organs as the brain and lungs.

PARONYCHIA OR "FELON"

Nature of the Condition

This is a specialized type of abscess that occurs at the junction of the fingernail and the cuticle. It is almost always associated with nail or cuticle biting or picking.

Symptoms

All symptoms of an abscess are present: pain, redness, swelling, and usually in a day or two, pus. When the pus is still under tension, prior to rupture of the abscess, the tip of the finger may be throbbingly painful. After the abscess ruptures, the pain diminishes and a crust forms.

Occasionally, the abscess circles all around the cuticle—both sides plus the bottom. This is called a "runaround."

Usually, healing is spontaneous, but in some cases infection spreads to the deeper tissues of the finger or hand. This can be most serious and disabling.

Treatment and Role of the School Nurse

At all stages, antibiotic ointment, usually bacitracin, should be applied and the area covered by an adhesive bandage. Sometimes the infection heals without formation of pus.

Prior to formation of free pus, applying hot compresses or soaking the finger in a glass of warm water relieves pain and accelerates healing.

After the formation of pus, it may be necessary to refer the child to the physician so the abscess can be drained by gently inserting a sharp blade between the cuticle and the nail.

If the whole tip of the finger is red and swollen, emergency referral to a physician is mandatory with followup to make sure the parent complies.

Only in rare circumstances should a school nurse attempt drainage with a scalpel blade. If a physician is not available and the school nurse is expected to perform this procedure, there should have been adequate prior instruction and signed standing orders.

BOILS (FURUNCLES)

Nature of the Condition

A furuncle (feẃ-rung-kl) is the medical term for a skin abscess or boil. The infection usually starts below the skin and expands. The deeper below the skin that the infection begins, the larger the boil will be when it reaches the surface. Skin abscesses vary in size from one centimeter to the size of a golf ball.

Causes include insect bites or puncture wounds, like slivers, that deposit germs below the skin surface. These are usually fairly small. Occasionally, germs are deposited under the skin of a child who has a bloodstream infection. These are apt to be larger, and the child will be very ill and will rarely be in school.

Symptoms

The average boil is about ½ to 1 inch in diameter.

1. Initially there will only be pain with minimal swelling and redness at the site of the boil.
2. Within one day the redness and swelling will increase as will the pain.
3. Either that day or the next the center of the boil will begin to show a pale yellow color indicating pus formation.
4. The yellow area enlarges, becomes soft to the touch, and may drain spontaneously.
5. In larger abscesses that do not drain properly, the pus gradually gets thick and waxy so that when drainage finally does occur, the pus is apt to come out in one lump. This is known as a *core.*

Treatment

1. Prior to the abscess becoming fluctuant and purulent (soft with pus), warm applications and an antibiotic ointment such as bacitracin should be applied and covered with a padded protective dressing.

2. When the abscess is at the proper stage, the child should be referred to a doctor to have it opened with a sharp scalpel, not with a needle. Needle openings are too small; they are apt to close before enough pus drains out, and the abscess does not heal properly.

3. Antibiotic ointment should be applied for another day or two until healing is well under way.

4. Don't squeeze the abscess to try to express the core; most abscesses do not have one. In addition to causing needless pain, hard squeezing spreads the infection under the skin and delays healing.

Role of the School Nurse

1. Proper diagnosis and determining appropriate treatment relative to the stage of the abscess is well within the province of the school nurse.

2. Application of warm packs, bacitracin ointment, and protective dressings are appropriate.

3. Rarely should a school nurse lance or otherwise surgically open an abscess with a scalpel or needle. Exactly the same procedures apply as described for paronychia.

4. Warn others about the dangers of squeezing a boil.

ACNE

Nature of the Condition

Since about 85 percent of high school children have some degree of acne, it scarcely needs lengthy description. It is usually most severe in girls between ages fourteen and seventeen and in boys between ages sixteen and nineteen. It usually begins to subside at about age twenty-two.

It is caused by the action of androgens (male hormones) upon the sebaceous (wax) glands of the skin. The adrenal glands of both boys and girls secrete small amounts of androgen. However, acne is usually worse in boys because the testicles secrete large amounts of androgens during puberty. The sebaceous glands are found in the largest number in the skin of the face, chest, and back. These skin glands secrete sebum or wax, and when they over-react to hormonal stimulation, "whiteheads" or "blackheads" occur. The medical term for these blemishes is *comedo* (pronounced "kah-meh-doe").

A whitehead is a closed comedo and cannot drain out onto the skin surface. It slowly enlarges and bursts out of its capsule under the surrounding skin, gets secondarily infected, and causes a small pimple or abscess (boil). The deeper the original breakout, the larger the boil becomes before it finally ruptures out onto the skin surface or, occasionally, heals without rupturing. In either case, if the abscess is large enough, scarring results.

A blackhead is an open comedo that easily drains out onto the skin surface and rarely causes abscesses. The blackened tip is not from dirt or poor hygiene; it is the result of a combination of dead skin cells and skin pigment.

Symptoms

1. *Mild:* The disease is limited to open comedones (blackheads), closed comedones (whiteheads), and occasional small pimples. The lesions are found mainly on the face with a smaller number on the chest and back.

2. *Moderate:* In addition to comedones, pimples, small nodules (hard lumps), and abscesses appear. The shoulders, back and chest are most involved. The lesions on the face are more numerous. Healing lesions remain red for a long time, but eventually the normal skin color returns.

3. *Severe:* The abscesses are larger, more widespread, and often confluent with several small ones joining to form a large one. There is more reddish discoloration. The larger abscesses heal by scarring and leave a pitted, irregular skin surface.

Emotional Problems

A student with a single pimple is self-conscious. A teenager with moderate to severe acne feels severely socially handicapped. Students do not initiate discussions about these concerns, so they may not know that methods exist to alleviate their problems.

Modern treatment offers many new, effective medications. However, successful therapy requires careful and sustained patient cooperation. Support and encouragement by the school nurse can be a key factor in a student's continuing therapy and eventual recovery.

Treatment

1. *Topical therapy (ointments, lotions, and liquids on the skin surface).* Most cases can be successfully managed by this method alone. There are innumerable medicines available; some are beneficial, some of no value, and some are actually dangerous. The older medications usually contain varying combinations of sulfur and salicylic acid. They are usually safe but only minimally effective.

The newer medications consist of benzoyl peroxide and vitamin A acid (retinoic acid, tretinoin). They are used singly or in combination and must be applied with careful attention to detail to avoid untoward skin irritation (redness and peeling).

There is now good evidence that some of these medications in oral or topical form may cause birth defects. Pregnant schoolgirls need to be especially cautious. All medications should be used under a physician's supervision. There are many over-the-counter remedies and home remedies for acne. Most are harmless but give little or no help. Those containing mercury should never be used.

2. *Oral antibiotics.* The most commonly used oral antibiotic is tetracycline, though others have been used. They are only available when prescribed by a physician and require prolonged usage. They are only used in cases with many pustules and abscesses. Antibiotics can have significant adverse side effects, so careful followup and patient cooperation are necessary. With newer topical medications, oral antibiotics are not used as much as in the past.

3. *Diet.* For years many foods were thought to cause acne. Sweets, milk, shellfish, fatty foods, ice cream, and chocolate—the arch villain of all—have been implicated. We now know that hot dogs, hamburgers, and candy do not cause acne, nor do they aggravate it. While it is

certainly wise for those with a known food sensitivity to eliminate that food from their diet, it is now generally recognized by leading skin specialists that no food, even chocolate, causes or worsens acne. Nevertheless, beliefs about the effects of food persist so strongly that it can be counterproductive to try to dissuade some people. If a school nurse encounters a child on any bizarre and obviously unhealthful diet, she should definitely intervene through the principal, counselor, parent, or doctor.

4. *Other methods*

   a. Estrogens (female hormones)—for girls over 16 with severe acne; potentially serious side effects; occasional good results; careful medical supervision required.

   b. Oral zinc—no proven benefit; potentially serious side effects; to be avoided.

   c. Acne surgery—draining of abscesses, comedo removal; helpful if done skillfully.

   d. Intralesional therapy—injection of steroids into larger lesions; helpful if done skillfully.

   e. Phototherapy—ultraviolet light; value debatable; dangerous if overdone.

   f. X-ray—used frequently in the past, rarely used today; dangerous.

   g. Cryotherapy—freezing of skin with powdered dry-ice slush; requires skilled dermatologist; potential for burn and scar.

   h. Scar removal with acid or dermabrasion—for healed, old, severe scars; occasional good results if done skillfully.

   i. Oral vitamin A in large doses—of no benefit; usually harmful.

   j. Washing of face with cold water, alcohol, or special soaps—psychologically beneficial; rarely harmful; no benefit. Cleanliness is not the problem.

School Relevance and Role of the School Nurse

It is important for principals, coaches, and counselors to be aware of the psychological and emotional factors which accompany acne and also to remain aware of the following considerations.

1. *Physical education.* Some children, especially girls, have severe acne on the chest, shoulders, and back. They should not be forced to "suit-up" if they strongly object. They are usually willing to express their feelings to a female counselor or school nurse.

2. *Extracurricular activities.* Students with severe acne often need extra encouragement to attend school picnics, pep rallies, dances, and so on. Principals, counselors, and school nurses can play an active role.

3. *Compliance with medication.* Since treatment continues for months or years, and since adolescence is the rebellious period of life, it is common for children with acne not to follow doctors' orders. School nurses, by helping to elevate the students' morale and encouraging and complimenting the students' improved appearance, can motivate improved medication and treatment compliance.

4. *Coordination with physician.* Many acne patients receive physician-prescribed medication. Reports from the school nurse regarding improvement or worsening of the skin or adverse medicine reaction is helpful to the doctor.

5. *Counseling regarding diet and over-the-counter medications.* The school nurse must make sure the student is not using harmful lotions, creams, or liquids. Although the diet should be sensible and well balanced—a properly made hamburger or hot dog can be a complete meal—the school nurse should remain aware that diet plays no role in acne. Parents sometimes think that acne must be outlived, so they do not seek help. The school nurse can open the door to modern medical therapy through rap sessions or formal classes.

HERPES SIMPLEX

Nature of the Condition

This condition, also called fever blisters, is caused by the *herpes simplex* virus, of which there are two types.

Type I is most apt to occur around the lips and nose but can also occur in other facial and body areas. It is extremely common in children; tests show that 70 to 90 percent of adults have had it at some time in their lives. (See Figure 2–1.)

Type II is most apt to occur in the genital area and is one of the most common sexually transmitted diseases. (See Section 8, Venereal Disease.)

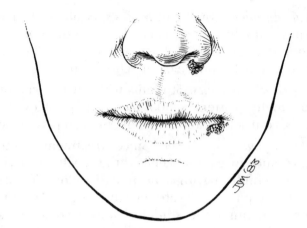

Figure 2–1. Some typical locations of herpes simplex

Symptoms

The active sore is the well-known, small fever blister seen on the lip. When the external sore heals, usually in six to ten days, the virus remains latent in the nerve trunks and may be reactivated following excess sunlight, fever, menstruation, and various other forms of physical or emotional stress.

The incubation period for either type of herpes varies from two to twelve days after exposure. Symptoms usually begin with a burning, tingling, or itching sensation at the site where the characteristic sores later appear. Generalized symptoms such as fever, malaise, sore throat, and headache can accompany the initial sores, which generally last no more than three weeks; after healing, no scars remain.

Recurrent sores tend to be less severe than the initial infection and persist for a shorter period of time, about four and a half days. Some children have no recurrent outbreaks while others may experience several recurrences per year.

Modes of Transmission

Both types of herpes are only contagious when the active lesions are present on the skin, *not* during the latent period when the virus is in the nerve trunks.

Type I is usually transmitted by direct contact with infected saliva or the active herpetic lesion itself, while type II is transmitted primarily through sexual contact. As in impetigo, autoinoculation of either type from active lesions on the lips or genitals to other body sites is possible. Since the virus can survive only a short time outside the body, it is unlikely that herpes could be contracted from toilet seats, hot tubs, or other inanimate objects.

Treatment

Currently, there is no medical treatment proven to be completely effective against genital or oral herpes; therefore, medical management should focus on symptomatic relief of pain and discomfort. To enhance healing and prevent secondary infection, the patient should clean the affected area with warm water and soap and dry it thoroughly.

Various ointments and lotions have been used with some unsubstantiated claims of success; aloe vera and Campho-Phenique are two of the more common. These are not harmful. Topical application of chloroform and ether have been recommended. They both sting but are not otherwise harmful.

Steroid ointments should not be used. Antibiotic ointments help only if there is secondary bacterial infection.

The latest medication which has been shown to accelerate healing in genital herpes is acyclovir (Zovirax). It comes in capsule and ointment form. It does not prevent recurrences. It is a new antiviral drug, requires a doctor's prescription and followup, and may have adverse side effects.

Prevention

It is important for herpes patients to be careful when handling their lesions to avoid the possibility of transferring the infection to other parts of their bodies. Patients should always wash their hands thoroughly after touching herpes sores. A disposable napkin or paper towel should be used to dry an area where lesions are present. Individuals who wear contact lenses should be particularly conscientious so as not to transmit the virus to their eyes. Anyone with active oral herpes lesions showing on their skin should avoid kissing or fondling others, especially newborn infants.

School Relevance and Role of the School Nurse

Many children will come to school with fever blisters (herpes simplex type I). They should not be excluded any more than a child with a common cold, but they should be privately counseled about hand cleanliness and should abstain from close-contact sports such as wrestling.

The nurse's most important function is to allay fears among school personnel and parents. There is a great deal of scare literature available today so people are apt to forget that children have been getting fever blisters for years. It is helpful to collect statements and other educational materials from the local health department.

Both types of herpes virus, I and II, are spread only by contact that is not likely to occur at school. The nurse should advise the principal that disinfecting the classrooms or the bathroom is of no value.

If children with herpes develop multiple lesions around the lips and nose, and especially on the fingertips, they are likely to have some secondary infection and will respond favorably to the application of antibiotic ointment two or three times a day.

Herpes simplex is one of a group of viruses that may be transmitted to the fetus, usually during delivery. (See Section 8).

SECTION 3

DISEASES OF THE EARS, NOSE, AND THROAT

The Common Cold
- Nature of the Condition and Diagnosis
- School Relevance and Role of the School Nurse
- Treatment

Colds vs. Nasal Allergy

Complications of Common Colds
- Middle Ear Infections
  - —Acute Otitis Media
  - —Serous Otitis Media
- Tonsil and Adenoid Infection
  - —Cause, Symptoms, and Diagnosis
  - —Treatment
- The Dilemma of Tonsillectomy
- Sinusitis
  - —Symptoms
  - —Treatment

THE COMMON COLD

Nature of the Condition and Diagnosis

In medical parlance, a common cold is a viral infection that begins with a runny nose and scratchy throat. Since the lining of the nose joins that of the sinuses, almost everybody with a cold has a certain degree of sinusitis also, even though they may not have any recognizable sinus symptoms. What we call a cold can be caused by some fifty to sixty different types and strains of viruses, each of which causes a slightly different set of symptoms. Some examples are:

1. A one- to three-day runny nose, with no other symptoms, that goes away rapidly and completely.
2. A seven- to fourteen-day runny nose with a slight sore throat and a little cough. There may be a low-grade fever the first day or two. The nasal secretions start clear and runny and gradually thicken and become greenish in color.
3. Same as 2 above, with some hoarseness caused by extension of the virus to the larynx (voice box).

With all of the above, the patient may have a little fever the first day or two, a slight feeling of malaise, and some loss of appetite.

4. Similar symptoms but with more fever, ranging from 102 to 104 degrees Fahrenheit in children and 100 to 102 degrees Fahrenheit in adults. This type of cold is the one that causes the most concern and may be associated with some secondary infection requiring specific treatment with antibiotics.

All colds are more common in children than in adults. Having a cold usually leaves some immunity to that particular virus, but since there are many others, it takes many years to develop a substantial immunity to the majority of respiratory viruses. Many children seem to catch one cold after another or to have a cold all winter long, especially after they start school or day care. Colds are also more severe in children, usually last longer, and cause higher fever and more complications.

School Relevance and Role of the School Nurse

Children continue to attend school with colds. Obviously, they are quite contagious, but it would be folly to try to keep all children with colds at home—the schools would be half-empty. Children are not harmed by attending school with a cold, provided they do not have fever and do not feel sick.

Treatment

Cold medications do not seem to alter the course of the disease, though they are usually harmless and may make the child more comfortable.

1. Acetaminophen (Tylenol) and similar types of medication are the most widely used medications for low-grade fevers and general malaise. They are safe if used in moderation. Aspirin is no longer recommended because of Reye's Syndrome. (See Section 8.) Many doctors believe that fever is a natural body mechanism which helps combat infections.

2. Nose drops may be necessary; however, a child may experience the negative effects of a rebound reaction which leaves the nose more stopped up than before. Nose drops are advisable only if used in moderation and for short periods.

3. There are two types of cough medicines. One type is an expectorant, which loosens the secretions and makes it easier to cough. This can relieve dry, hacking coughs which may be very troublesome. A child who cannot rest because of a continuous severe cough may require the second type—a sedative cough medicine. This type usually contains codeine or related substances which can be helpful if used properly. Because of their nature and mode of action, the sedative cough medicines usually require a prescription and should be used only under a doctor's guidance. If a cough is sedated too much, the retained excess secretions may lead to pneumonia.

The cough is nature's way of clearing undesirable secretions from the respiratory passages and, as such, is beneficial. If the cough does not excessively bother the child, it is not necessary to do anything about it at all. One can be reassured that through coughing, secretions are being forced up out of the lungs and bronchial tubes. Parents as well as teachers often worry because children swallow these secretions. But this is what nature intended; it does no harm whatsoever.

There are dozens of so-called remedies on the market today, and many people are convinced that they help—about as many are convinced that they don't help. Most of them contain varying combinations of acetaminophen, an antihistamine, and an occasional decongestant.

My personal philosophy is, "the less medicine the better." Children who are not excessively uncomfortable should be left alone for one or two weeks to get well by themselves. If some of the symptoms (cough or runny nose) cause particular discomfort, follow the recommendations of the doctor or school nurse.

COLDS VS. NASAL ALLERGY

A cold is an acute respiratory infection that begins, runs its course, and ends. It lasts from two or three to fourteen days, depending on the virus. At onset the nasal secretions are thin and clear and gradually get thicker before going away.

Allergies, on the other hand, last a full season, usually spring or fall, or quite commonly all year. The secretions usually stay thin and clear. A cough is less likely to develop, though sneezing can be severe. The child usually does not feel bad or have fever.

Unfortunately, many children with nasal allergy get colds more easily and more often than nonallergic children, so they present a mixed picture of a cold implanted on an allergic nasal mucus membrane (inner lining). When this happens, the child who has a runny nose all year will begin to feel bad, perhaps develop a little fever, and often develop a cough. In many cases, even for a physician, it's very difficult to tell one from the other.

COMPLICATIONS OF COMMON COLDS

Middle Ear Infections

Acute Otitis Media

Symptoms and Diagnosis

A middle ear infection (*otitis media*) is usually a complication of a cold. The younger the child, the greater the incidence of otitis media. By school age, this complication becomes less common than in babies and toddlers. *Acute otitis media typically begins with high fever and earache.*

Treatment and School Action

This complication always requires treatment by a physician because specific antibiotics are usually needed. Most doctors prescribe treatment for seven to fourteen days. The child usually feels pretty well after the first day or two and may return to school. The antibiotic needs to be continued, however, and it is often given four times a day. This means that on a schedule of 8:00 A.M., 12:00 P.M., 4:00 P.M., and 8:00 P.M., one dose must be given at school. School authorities should always allow this medication to be given by the school nurse or other assigned person because relapses are very common if otitis is not treated diligently enough. Repeated relapses may cause some degree of hearing loss, which proper treatment usually prevents.

Many doctors now believe that otitis media can be treated just as effectively by giving the oral antibiotic three times a day: at about breakfast (6:30-8:00), return from school (3:30-4:00), and at bedtime (8:00-10:00). This schedule obviates the need for a dose at school, most children and parents prefer this, and I recommend it.

Serous Otitis Media

Symptoms and Diagnosis

An acute inflammation of the middle ear usually causes fever and earache, but with proper treatment the patient gets well completely, in which case the middle ear and the ear drum return to pre-illness normality. However, serous otitis media (SOM) (also called otitis media with effusion—OME) is a frequent complication. In this condition, a small collection of serum (straw colored, thin, watery fluid derived from blood plasma) fills the middle ear cavity and causes a small hearing loss. This fluid collection usually *does not cause pain* or other symptoms. The effusion usually is absorbed and disappears by itself in one to three weeks but occasionally it persists, and the fluid thickens and may impede the mobility of the ear drum. This can cause permanent, mild conductive hearing loss. Proper medical management can prevent this complication; antibiotics and a small incision in the ear drum to drain the fluid are usually sufficient. Occasionally a tympanotomy tube must be inserted.

The same disease process, OME, can occur following a common cold even when there is no acute ear infection with its accompanying earache or fever. Without these symptoms, the condition is apt to be overlooked, since the child is not aware of any hearing loss and does not complain of pain.

Treatment and School Action

Comparison with an audiogram previous to the OME would show a present mild conductive loss in the ear with the effusion. The loss will be small, 30–50 dB, and equal across all frequencies.

Obviously, the nurse cannot do an audiogram on all children with a common cold, but for a child who is recuperating from an acute middle ear infection, the teacher should be alerted to the possibility of hearing loss and the need for an audiogram.

If the audiogram shows a mild conductive loss, the child should not be referred to the doctor unless the hearing loss persists for three weeks. Most middle ear effusions resolve spontaneously in that period of time.

Tonsil and Adenoid Infection

Cause, Symptoms and Diagnosis

In addition to the large, red, painful tonsils, the glands (lymph nodes) in the neck become swollen and tender. The adenoids usually get infected at the same time. This is usually a complication of a cold, though sometimes the runny nose and cough follow the sore throat and fever.

Tonsillitis can be caused by a strep throat (a streptococcus germ); a throat culture is required to identify it. Some school nurses do throat cultures in the school clinic using a rapid test kit. Two that are reliable are "Culturette" and "Directogen." They can be ordered from American Scientific Products, 210 Great S.W. Parkway, Grand Prairie, TX 78050.

Treatment

Untreated, a strep infection can lead to rheumatic fever with subsequent severe heart damage. Sufficient and correctly chosen antibiotics will prevent this complication. Referral to a doctor is always necessary for bacterial cultures and clinical judgment to determine the correct antibiotic to use.

The Dilemma of Tonsillectomy

Whether or not to remove tonsils is a complicated decision that only an experienced and conscientious physician can properly resolve. This is one of the most commonly over-performed operations, so much so that some insurance companies will pay for a consultant in an attempt to reduce the number. On the other hand, there are certain children for whom tonsillectomy is essential:

1. Recurrent tonsillitis, to the extent that the child fails to grow and thrive and misses school once or twice every month for two to five days, despite adequate antibiotics. This child often does exceptionally well after surgery.

2. Frequent middle ear infections. Otitis media is often associated with tonsillitis. Persistent ear infections that do not respond to medication can result in permanent hearing loss. In these cases, tonsil and/or adenoid removal must be considered.

3. Severe mouth breathing that actually causes the child to be noticeably odd-looking, have some difficulty in swallowing, and snore loudly at night. These children are usually underweight and sickly because of chronic tonsillar infection and are easily susceptible to all infections.

4. Other rare severe conditions, such as peritonsillar abscess.

About twenty-five to thirty years ago, doctors felt that most chilen would do better without tonsils and adenoids. As time went by, it was realized that most of this surgery was unnecessary and that there were significant surgical risks and complications. The pendulum swung so far the other way that some children who really needed their tonsils and adenoids removed were denied surgery, especially by younger doctors who were trained in accordance with the newer medical beliefs and who had not had time to see the deleterious effects of long-term tonsillitis. At the present time, there is a good bit of research being carried out to try to define the exact conditions that require surgical removal as opposed to antibiotic treatment. In the meantime, the only safe course is to follow the doctor's advice, but be wary of a too casual suggestion for removal of tonsils and adenoids or a suggestion that the doctor might as well do two or three children in the same family at the same time. In case of doubt, another doctor, preferably an experienced pediatrician, should be consulted. Responsible doctors do not resent a request for consultation.

Sinusitis

Symptoms

Although the sinuses are always somewhat invoved in any cold, in certain cases the cold seems to settle in the sinuses. In these cases, the secretions become thick and greenish-yellow; the cough becomes more prominent and is especially pronounced in the morning. During the night, the secretions collect in the upper air passages after draining from the sinuses into the nose and down the throat. Headache is common, usually over the eyes, but sometimes involving the entire head and increasing in the afternoon. The cough may last a long time, occasionally all winter.

Treatment

Treatment takes a long time. Decongestants, antihistamines, nose drops, and antibiotics are all used for different types of sinusitis. Vaporizers may provide symptomatic relief at night. The long-term outlook is good. Most individuals get completely well, but occasionally, people with nasal allergies develop chronic sinusitis which may last several years.

SECTION 4

EYE PROBLEMS

Glossary of Eye Terminology
- School Relevance

Refractive Errors
- Hyperopia
- Myopia
- Astigmatism

Amblyopia
- Nature of the Condition
- Treatment

Conjunctivitis
- Nature of the Condition
- Treatment
- Role of the School Nurse

Contact Lenses
- Types of Contact Lenses
- • Lens Cleaning Procedure
  —Amoeba Infections
- Instructions for Proper Use of Contact Lenses
- Instructions for When the Lens is Out of Position

Eye Strain
- Adequate Lighting

GLOSSARY OF EYE TERMINOLOGY

An ophthalmologist, or eye doctor, follows procedures and practices that are highly specialized, more so than in almost any other specialty of medicine. Therefore, an alphabetical glossary is included here to help you understand the unique but necessary vocabulary that describes the abnormalities eye specialists see and the procedures they perform. This little "eye dictionary" should help the school nurse understand the ophthalmologist's report and some of the reasoning behind what the doctor suggests.

Accommodation. Contraction of the ciliary muscle causing the lens to become rounder and therefore thicker. This causes light rays entering the eye to be used for close reading.

Amblyopia. Blindness of an eye caused by disuse; also called *amblyopia exanopsia* or *lazy eye*.

Anisometropia. A difference in the refractive index of the eyes causing double or blurred vision unless one eye is closed or unless vision in one eye is subconsciously suppressed by the brain. This can cause amblyopia also.

Astigmatism. Abnormal shape of the lens (rare) or the cornea (clear center of the eyeball) causing blurred vision.

Conjunctivitis. Irritation or inflammation of the thin layer of transparent skin covering the eyeball and inner surface of the eyelids.

Convergence. Both eyes pointing toward the nose simultaneously. This occurs automaticaly during reading or looking at close objects.

Cross-eye. One or both eyes permanently deviating inward.

Diplopia. Double vision. The child will tend to see two blurred objects rather than one clearly defined image.

Divergence. Both eyes deviating away from the nose simultaneously.

Esophoria. One or both eyes deviating toward the nose only in special circumstances—if the child is tired, gazing into the distance, or under certain testing conditions.

Esotropia. See *cross-eye*.

Exophoria. Same as *esophoria* but with deviation away from the nose.

Exotropia. One or both eyes permanently deviating away from the nose.

Hyperopia. Farsightedness. The eyeball is shorter than normal, light focuses behind the retina, and vision is blurred.

Myopia. Nearsightedness. The eyeball is longer than normal, light focuses in front of the retina, and vision is blurred.

Phoria. A generic term meaning a tendency for either eye to deviate inward or outward.

Pinkeye. See *conjunctivitis.*

Strabismus. Any condition in which the two eyes do not fuse properly and look at the same object at the same time. Also called squint because lack of proper fusion causes *diplopia* so the child closes one eye to see clearly.

Tropia. A generic term meaning that either eye actually does deviate inward or outward most or all of the time.

School Relevance

As long as a child is performing well in school and has no complaints, it is usually correctly assumed that the eyes are normal. (See Figure 4–1.) However, as soon as an average child begins to fall

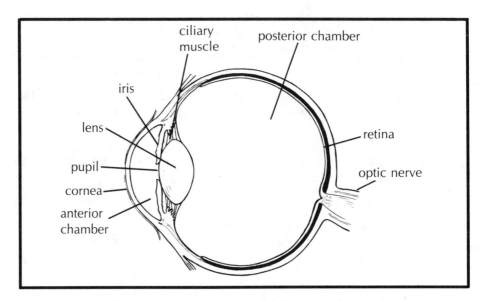

Figure 4–1. Cross-section of the Normal Eye.

behind in schoolwork, one of the first things that occurs to the teacher is to have the eyes (vision) checked, and the eye doctor's report is often difficult to interpret. The best time to check a child's eyes is at age three. Some school nurses and teachers see three-year-old children and should be on the alert for any evidence that a child favors one eye over the other.

REFRACTIVE ERRORS

There are three kinds of refractive errors. They are hyperopia, myopia, and astigmatism. (See Figure 4–2.)

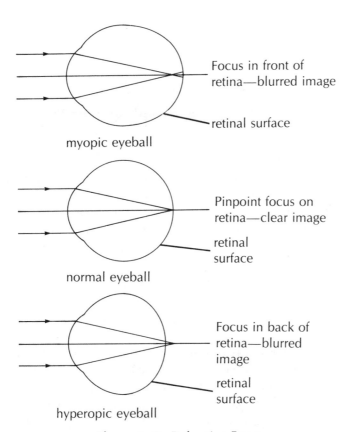

Figure 4–2. Refractive Errors

Hyperopia

In farsightedness (*hyperopia*) distant vision is better than close vision. In mild cases, distant vision is normal and only a small amount of accommodation during reading is required to cause the light to focus slightly farther in front and fall exactly on the retina; glasses are not needed. In moderate cases, distant vision may also be normal, but the child, in order to achieve clear vision while reading close, must accommodate so much that eyestrain develops. This can cause headache, eye pain, fatigue, nausea, and disinclination to read. In severe cases, distant vision is blurred unless strong accommodating efforts are made, and clear vision for reading is impossible. On occasion, reading matter is held close to the nose. Glasses are necessary for the child with moderate to severe hyperopia.

Myopia

Nearsightedness (*myopia*) means close vision is better than distant vision. It exists in varying degrees of severity also, but glasses are always necessary because the light rays already focus in front of the retina and accommodating efforts would merely focus the rays farther in front. Myopic children cannot see distant objects clearly but do not know it (never having had normal vision). The problem is often first discovered during school screening examinations. These children usually hold reading material very close to their noses to be able to see clearly and often squint or frown to see better. This can cause the same symptoms as in hyperopia.

Astigmatism

In cases of astigmatism, vision is blurred at any distance. Caused by an irregularly shaped cornea, astigmatism cannot be influenced by accommodation, so glasses are necessary. Holding reading matter close to the eyes, squinting, and frowning are also seen in moderate to severe degrees of astigmatism.

AMBLYOPIA

Nature of the Condition

Children who do not see equally with both eyes will have double vision. This is so uncomfortable and distracting that these children will rapidly and subconsciously suppress vision in the poorer eye, learn to use only the better eye, and grow up with an eye that is blind because it has never developed a functional connection with the visual centers of the brain. It takes about seven years for the nerve tracts that connect the eye to the back of the brain to fully develop, and the eyes must be used during this development. If vision has not developed by age seven, there is no chance that it will develop later. This type of blindness is called amblyopia, or lazy eye. (See Section 17, Vision Screening.)

There are two principal abnormalities that cause amblyopia, *strabismus* and *anisometropia*. Strabismus—when the two eyes do not fuse properly to look at an object—is by far the more common of these conditions. Anisometropia is a difference in refractive power in the two eyes. For example, if one eye is hyperopic and the other is myopic, the hyperopic eye will develop amblyopia if not treated. It is said that the overall incidence of anisometropia is 0.5 to 1.0 percent of all children. It is usually discovered in screening programs; a child may see 20/40 with one eye and 20/20 with the other.

Treatment

Once amblyopia is fully established, restoration of vision is impossible. Prevention consists of diagnosing the precursory conditions—strabismus or anisometropia—at a young enough age. If treatment is begun by the age of three, almost all amblyopia can be prevented. With each year of advancing age, the amount of vision remaining becomes less and less, so that by age six or seven permanent blindness has already developed in the amblyopic eye.

From the above discussion, it is easy to see the importance of preschool eye-screening programs. All three-year-old children of average intelligence can be given a reliable vision exam with simple screening tests. Certainly, any child with a squint, abnormal eye movements, or other unusual visual habits should be seen by an eye doctor.

CONJUNCTIVITIS

Nature of the Condition

Conjunctivitis is an inflammation of the thin, transparent outer layer of the eyeball and the inner surface of the eyelids. The inflammation causes redness, tearing, and occasionally formation of pus. Because of the redness, it is commonly called pinkeye, and the most common causes are bacteria, viruses, and allergy. The first two are quite contagious. Allergic conjunctivitis is usually associated with nasal allergy and rarely causes any pus in the inner corner of the eye; this can be helpful in differentiating contagious from noncontagious varieties.

Treatment

Bacterial conjunctivitis is the cause of about 55 to 65 percent of cases of pinkeye. Treatment usually consists of antibiotic eye drops or ointments, and most cases heal very quickly. However, if the infectious conjunctivitis is caused by a virus, antibiotic drops will not help. Therefore, some children with mild pinkeye will be told by their physician that no treatment is necessary, and the condition will go away by itself in a few days.

Allergic conjunctivitis can be relieved, not cured, by certain nonantibiotic eye drops.

There are no longer any eye drops manufactured in the U.S. that contain mercury, but some may still be available over-the-counter in foreign countries. Some people develop serious reactions to mercury.

Role of the School Nurse

If new cases of pinkeye occur at two-week intervals, they are probably not related, because the incubation period is only three to five days. Each case should be evaluated by the school nurse. If the pinkeye appears infectious, it should be referred to a physician; if allergic, it can be observed for a day or two to see if it goes away. If no medication is prescribed, the child should be observed daily; if the condition worsens, the doctor or parent should be notified.

When new cases begin to occur daily, it is important to remove each infected child from the campus as soon as possible to contain the epidemic. Although most pinkeye is contagious, it is not always medically necessary to exclude children from school for more than a day. Common colds are also contagious, and we do not insist that children with colds stay home. In such situations, school nurses should base their decisions on the above criteria.

CONTACT LENSES

Many school children are now wearing contact lenses which often cause eye problems because the children either do not know how to exercise the proper care required to wear contacts, or they are too young to feel vulnerable when they break the rules. The wonder is that more do not have serious eye disease, judging by how many children wash their lenses in their mouths.

Types of Contact Lenses

1. Hard, remove each night
   a. Traditional: nonpermeable
   b. Newer: gas (oxygen) permeable. These lenses can be worn longer each day without discomfort. They are slightly more expensive and require more meticulous care than the nonpermeable.

2. Soft, remove each night. When wet, these lenses are soft and supple; when dry they are rigid and fragile. They must be kept moist at all times.
   • Comfortable almost immediately
   • Last about eighteen months
   • Ideal for athletes
   • Require meticulous care and weekly sterilization
3. Soft, extended wear. These lenses are especially designed to be worn for one week to three months. They require motivated wearers who will care for them meticulously and comply with their doctors' orders.

Important Facts

Myopia is not corrected by contact lenses. The hard lenses do tend to flatten the cornea slightly and thus improve myopic vision, but this is temporary; the cornea resumes its previous shape after the lenses are removed.

In sports, soft contacts are safest. Hard lenses, however, pose no greater dangers than do regular glasses.

For severe myopia and astigmatism, hard contacts are better than soft.

Lens Cleaning Procedure

Regardless of which type of lens is used, cleaning and disinfecting the lenses are important.

Cleaning: Cleaning is done first with a salt or enzyme solution which removes impurities which build up on the lens.

Disinfecting: Disinfection, which is usually done with a chemical solution (as opposed to heat sterilization), is sufficient to kill most germs, but may not kill all germs capable of causing a corneal infection.

Amoeba Infections

Recently there have been increasing reports of an eye infection caused by an amoeba which is abundant in soil and water. It has even been found in nonsterile distilled water, which some wearers use to clean lenses. This infection is particularly serious because no antibiotic will cure it and partial or complete blindness may result. It occurs most often in users of soft contact lenses which are not changed as frequently. Therefore, only commercially prepared sterile cleaning and disinfecting solutions should be used.

Instructions for Proper Use of Contact Lenses

- Never sleep with your lenses in place unless advised by the doctor (under special conditions) to do so.
- Do not use saliva as a "wetting" agent. The risk of bacterial contamination is great.
- Never rinse your lenses in hot water or store in an unusually hot or cold place as lense warpage may occur. Do not "flex" your lenses. This can also warp them.
- Eye make-up should be used sparingly around the eyelids.
- Avoid swimming when wearing contacts as they can easily be washed out and lost.
- If at any time you stop wearing your lenses for a few days, your corneas may lose their adaptation and you will need to restrict your wearing time for a short periods.
- Watch your "blinking habits." Good "blinking" is *essential* in all forms of contact lens wear. This keeps a constant fresh supply of oxygen to the corneas and helps to "wet" the lens surfaces.

Instructions for When the Lens Is Out of Position

Recentering the Lens

1. A lens may be left on the white of the eye indefinitely without injury or discomfort.
2. If movement of the lens seems very difficult, flood the area with drops of water and roll the eye.
3. The lens can be moved to different positions by manipulation through the lids.

4. If you become tense, a rest will restore your coordination, and a second try will succeed.

Lens Under Upper Lid

1. Look down with eyes.
2. With finger on upper lash margin, pull upper lid up and press against white of the eye.
3. Push lens down to center and hold.
4. Look straight ahead.

Lens Under Lower Lid

1. Look up with eyes.
2. With finger on lower margin, pull lower lid down and press against white of the eye.
3. Push lens up to center and hold.
4. Look straight ahead.

Lens in Outside Corner

1. Place thumb and first finger on lash margin near outside corner of eye.
2. Spread lids apart.
3. Look to your nose.
4. Push lens with lids to center and hold.
5. Look straight ahead.

Lens in Inside Corner

1. Place first finger of each hand on upper and lower lash margin.
2. Spread lids apart.
3. Look to outside corner toward ear.
4. Push lens with the lids to center and hold.
5. Look straight ahead.

EYE STRAIN

Adequate Lighting

How much light (usually measured in candlepower or lumens) should be present for adequate reading and writing? There is much literature on this subject, but most of it is less than scientific. The amount of light necessary for school children to perform academic tasks comfortably varies, but 50 lumens per square foot of reading surface is often considered optimal. A 60-watt incandescent bulb emits about 850 to 900 lumens. A 60-watt (four foot) fluorescent bar emits about 3300 to 4300 lumens. However, many children do quite well studying under 20 to 30 lumens per square foot for long periods. For shorter periods even 10 lumens reduces efficiency only 7 percent.

It is often stated that children reading with inadequately directed light or in dim light will develop eye strain. In actuality, children and adults with normal eyes, with or without glasses, can read quite comfortably in a wide range of candlepower and with light coming from a variety of sources. In general, if a teacher with normal eyes can read comfortably, he or she can rest assured that the students can also. In addition, there are no long- or short-range ill effects on the eyes if one reads for short periods with less than adequate lighting.

Recently there have been concerns about the types of light bulbs used. In the classroom, old-fashioned incandescent bulbs and both types of fluorescent bar bulbs—cool white and daylight—have proved to have no adverse effect on children. The two newer lights—sodium vapor which casts a yellowish light and mercury vapor which casts a bluish light—have been reported to cause stomach aches, headaches, nervousness, and other vague symptoms in some children. Therefore, they should be used only in open playgrounds and not in enclosed classrooms.

SECTION 5

DISEASES OF THE LUNGS

Asthma
- Nature of the Condition
- School Relevance
- Participation in Physical Education
- Physician Involvement
- Acute Asthmatic Emergencies
- Treatment
  —Prevention
  —Treatment of Acute Asthma
  —Teaching Children

Bronchitis
- Nature of the Condition and Symptoms
- Treatment and School Relevance

Pneumonia
- Nature of the Condition
- Symptoms
- School Relevance and Role of the School Nurse
- Treatment

Tuberculosis
- Nature of the Condition
- Treatment
- Contagiousness
- Tuberculin Skin Testing and School Attendance

Pleurisy

ASTHMA

Nature of the Condition

Asthma is an allergic disease of the lungs that causes constriction of the smaller bronchioles (small air passages). The typical attack causes moderate to severe difficulty in breathing. There is always some associated wheezing even though it may not be audible to the unaided ear. The children always experience some degree of distress and anxiety—the more severe the attack, the more anxious and worried they are.

In many cases, the allergic asthmatic attack is accompanied by an infection in the respiratory tract. When this occurs, the child has significant fever and may need antibiotics in addition to asthma medicine.

School Relevance

Asthma is one of the most common serious childhood illnesses that must be dealt with in school. It is rarely life-threatening, but it does in many cases affect a child's entire life-style. Children with moderately severe asthma miss school often, must visit the doctor frequently, make many trips to hospital emergency rooms, and have probably been hospitalized several times. They take a lot of medicine and get many shots. Also, they are socially limited. They come to be known as sickly and in time think of themselves that way. With all of this, it is easy to see why the disease has an effect far beyond the actual wheezing episode. Fortunately, most children "outgrow" their asthma. Attacks occur very frequently in preschool and elementary school children, but by middle school years they usually diminish in frequency and intensity.

Treatment is often necessary during the school day. The most common medicine prescribed is in an inhaler that must be used as soon as an attack begins. Many children carry their own medication in their pocket or purse. This practice may be at odds with a school district policy that requires all medication to be administered by a nurse or her designate. This dilemma should be resolved at the local school or district level. There are many reasons for each position; I prefer a case-by-case decision made by a conference with the parent, doctor, principal, and, if appropriate, the child.

Participation in Physical Education

Participation in sports is controversial. Until ten to fifteen years ago, doctors felt that children with asthma should not be overly active because running and playing usually exaggerate the coughing and wheezing. Children with a condition called *exercise-induced asthma* do not wheeze until they do something that makes them breathe fast. Hard laughing and running will bring on an attack.

Doctors, as well as parents, prefer that asthmatic children avoid activities known to bring on attacks. An overzealous physical education teacher may insist that all children exercise every day. Lest anybody point the finger at gym teachers for being cruel and heartless, it must be said that many doctors will write an excuse from gym for long periods (sometimes all year) on very flimsy grounds. In any case, teachers should know that some asthmatic children should limit exercise and for a certain period in their lives must forego the pleasures and benefits of active competitive sports. However, this does not in any way mean that asthma should preclude total participation in all sports. Relatively quieter sports such as archery or golf are salutory and maintain body tone without increasing the respiratory rate.

Most children with asthma are perfectly normal between attacks and should be allowed to exercise to the full limits of their tolerance. With the recent increased emphasis on physical fitness, jogging, and so on, it is current practice to recommend graded exercise for asthmatic children to enhance general body strength and muscle tone in the hope that they will get fewer attacks, be better able to withstand the attacks they do get, and generally lead a more happy and productive life. While this has not yet been proven, it seems reasonable.

Many children with asthma are overprotected by parents and doctors to the point that they themselves become convinced that any exercise will bring on an attack. Because of the emotional aspects of asthma, they are often correct. This type of child would probably be helped by graded and carefully monitored physical exercise. Unfortunately, there are few public schools in the United States that employ special adaptive physical education teachers to develop special programs for handicapped children. If encouraged to exercise without guidance, children will typically overexert themselves past their point of tolerance. Many adults, especially males, do the same thing when they enter an exercise program.

Physician Involvement

The child with asthma often ends up in the center of a triangle with parents at one corner, doctor at the other, and physical education teacher at the third. All too often they are not working cooperatively. The parents tend to be overprotective, the physical education teacher overdemanding, and the doctor too casual and unable (or unwilling) to understand the social and psychological implications of the school problem. To avoid such a situation, the doctor, parents, and physical education teacher—each respecting and understanding the other— should confer, discuss the situation rationally, and agree on a plan for the year. If this requires more time than they can give, a three-way telephone conference is a useful substitute. This problem usually arises in sixth or seventh grade, and by that time the methods of coping and the relationships between the child, the parents, and the doctor have been well established. If a child has a note from the doctor saying that he or she should be excused from physical education for the whole year because of asthma, teachers should not be too insistent on physical education participation. Refer the problem to the principal to deal with as an administrative matter. It is a mistake to equate physical fitness with total health. One or two years without physical education are not crucial in a child's lifetime, and most children outgrow their asthma (or most of it) by high school.

Acute Asthmatic Emergencies

The majority of asthmatic attacks that occur at school are controlled quickly by inhalant use. On rare occasion, the attack will not subside even when the inhaler is used properly, followed by the prescribed brief waiting period, and then used again. If the attack does not subside, the child will begin to get frightened and the anxiety will make the asthma even worse.

In this situation, if a parent cannot be immediately located to take the child to the doctor, the best course is immediate evacuation to a hospital emergency room by an emergency ambulance service or by the school nurse accompanied by a driver.

Treatment

Prevention

1. Allergy shots and removal of allergens.
2. Chromolyn is a medication that can be taken by inhaler to render the lining of the respiratory tracts less sensitive. An inhalation two to four times a day is often beneficial.
3. Theophyllin is a medication taken by mouth to dilate the bronchial tubes. It is sold under a number of trade names, for example, Slo-bid, Theodur, Elixophyllin, and Quibron. It is effective but may cause lightheadedness, poor attention span, poor memory, headache, poor behavior control, and other adverse side effects.
4. Steroids by mouth or inhaler have numerous adverse side effects and are used only in severe cases.

Treatment of Acute Attack

The most common treatment is the inhaler which puts out a fine mist of medicines generically called beta adrenergics. Some of their trade names are Proventil and Ventolin. These medications are related to adrenalin but are safer because they are slower acting.

Straight adrenalin is available in a mist form also. Its trade name is Primatene. It can be purchased without a prescription and is effective but dangerous because it is so quick acting. It may cause a sudden rise in blood pressure with, cardiac arrest in rare cases.

Needless to say, all medication should be given only under the direction of a physician, preferably an allergist. Each child's treatment must be individualized. Children should *never* share their medicine.

Teaching Children How to Take Their Medicine

Many children use their inhaler incorrectly; they put the end in their mouth, squeeze, and inhale. The proper method is to hold the end about 3 inches in front of the mouth, *exhale* as much air as possible, squeeze the inhaler and inhale the cloud of mist as deeply as possible. Always gently shake the inhaler before each use.

There are several books for children, parents and teachers; the following two are recommended:

- *Teaching Myself about Asthma,* Parcel, et al., St. Louis: C.V. Mosby, 1979.
- *Advancing Swiftly to the Healthy Management of Asthma*—1987 Vol. 1, K–3. Vol. 2, 4–6. Vol. 3, 7–9
  American Lung Association of Los Angeles
  5858 Wilshire Blvd.
  Los Angeles, CA 90036

BRONCHITIS

Nature of the Condition and Symptoms

Bronchitis is an infection of the bronchial tubes. These tubes carry the air down to the air sacs in the lungs where oxygen is absorbed into the bloodstream. This condition can follow a cold, and though the children usually feel well and have no fever, a troublesome cough persists for several weeks after the cold goes away. On a winter walk through the school halls it sometimes sounds like a small herd of walruses. The cough usually starts out "tight"—dry, hacking, and nonproductive of sputum. Later it gets looser, wetter, more productive, and less frequent. It often takes four to six weeks to go away. In some children with allergic bronchitis, the cough can last all winter.

Treatment and School Relevance

The only medicines available for this condition are cough medicines. They are not very effective in controlling the cough unless one gives relatively large doses of sedative cough medicines, and this can suppress the cough so much that dangerous amounts of secretions are retained in the lungs. The cough is almost always made worse by physical exertion, so it may help to limit physical education and/or recess. During the time when the cough is severe, though it sounds horrible, it is not very contagious. Whether or not children should stay home depends on how much the cough bothers the child and others.

PNEUMONIA

Nature of the Condition

Pneumonia is an infection of the air sacs of the lungs. In the past several years, many physicians have been using the word *pneumonitis* instead of pneumonia. Though the two words mean the same thing, it has become common practice to use pneumonitis when one means a small area of infection with minimal symptoms, and pneumonia for larger areas of infection with more severe symptoms.

Normal lungs are soft and spongy since they are filled with air. When a child develops pneumonia, the involved portion of the lung becomes very dense and consolidated.

The lungs are divided into separate portions called lobes—two on the left and three on the right. Infection of an entire lobe is called lobar pneumonia. When the infection involves smaller patches in one or several places simultaneously, it is called bronchopneumonia.

There are many different kinds of pneumonias. Acute lobar pneumonia with a very high fever can occur very suddenly and is still a formidable cause of death in many parts of the world. However, with proper diagnosis and treatment, it is usually one of the easiest diseases to cure. On the other hand, bronchopneumonia caused by certain types of viruses can be so mild that the child has only a mild cough and a very low-grade fever and is hardly sick. This very mild type is often referred to as *walking pneumonia*.

Symptoms

School nurses have reason to suspect pneumonia when the following symptoms are present:

1. *Cough.* Almost all children with pneumonia have some type of cough, the most common being a relatively small loose cough that is not overly troublesome.

2. *Fever.* High fever is present in most children but occasionally it will be low.

3. *Lassitude, loss of appetite, drowsiness, and general malaise.* These latter symptoms, of course, are common to almost all children's illnesses.

School Relevance and Role of the School Nurse

The child with frank pneumonia is usually quite sick and therefore will not be in school. Teachers and nurses, however, will see many children with a cough who may have a temperature of 100 degrees Fahrenheit to 100.6 degrees Fahrenheit orally. When these symptoms are combined with those listed in the third group above, it is wise to refer the child to a doctor, especially if, after a day or two, the child does not run and play as usual. Since pneumonia presents such a highly variable set of symptoms, it is not wise for a teacher, principal, or parent to wait too long before having the child examined.

While a few specific varieties of pneumonia are contagious, the types that are most often seen in school are not. Most pneumonia is caused by germs or viruses that are present in healthy children, and the children who actually develop disease in their lungs do so because of individual susceptibility—not by catching it from another child who may come to school with pneumonia.

Treatment

All children with pneumonia need a certain amount of rest. Almost all of them need antibiotics. The treatment should always be managed by a physician.

TUBERCULOSIS

Nature of the Condition

There are two types of *tuberculosis:* primary, usually occurring in childhood, and secondary, usually occurring in adults. The primary type represents the body's first encounter with the tuberculosis germ (*tubercle bacillus*). The infection localizes in the lymph nodes near the center of the lungs and in most cases is self-cured by normal body resistance. While there are no outwardly visible traces, an x-ray sometimes shows permanent evidence of healed tuberculosis. The incidence of primary tuberculosis is diminishing.

Primary tuberculosis triggers a change in the body's immune reaction mechanism. The entire body, including the skin, becomes allergic to the tubercle bacillus for many years thereafter. Therefore, if a tuberculin skin test is performed, it causes a typical reddish reaction. If the same skin test is performed on a person who has never had tuberculosis, it will cause no reaction. When a child first shows a positive skin test, it is necessary that he or she have a chest x-ray to make sure that the disease is not in its active stage. While most primary tuberculosis is mild and cures itself, an unusual case may require extensive treatment.

Treatment

Streptomycin, discovered in the mid-1940s, was the first medicine available to treat tuberculosis. Now it is reserved for certain rare and severe types. Most cases can be cured with several other oral medications.

As a precautionary standard practice, all persons under age thirty-five with a positive skin test are treated for one year, usually with INH (isonicotinic acid hydrazide) alone. This prevents any possibility of a severe and sometimes fatal complication that may follow childhood tuberculosis.

Contagiousness

Adult tuberculosis is contagious; the childhood type is not at all contagious. This paradox arises from the fact that children with childhood tuberculosis do not cough up tuberculosis germs. Childhood or primary tuberculosis settles in a part of the lung near the center and does not irritate the bronchial tubes; therefore, there is no cough to spread the germs into the air. Older children or teenagers, of course, may develop the adult type (secondary tuberculosis). If they do, they cough and are just as contagious as adults. Obviously, a doctor's advice is necessary to determine whether any individual child with tuberculosis is contagious or not.

Tuberculin Skin Testing and School Attendance

The prevalence of tuberculosis in the U.S. has been slowly decreasing for the past forty to fifty years. It is now so low that mass skin testing is done only in school districts that have a significant prevalence, mainly those that are near Mexico. If there is any question, direction should be taken from the local health department.

Children whose skin test is positive should be referred to their physician or to the local health authorities who will recommend appropriate treatment. Though fears among teachers and parents will often be generated when tests are found to be positive, these children are not contagious.

Many years ago, children with diagnosed tuberculosis had to miss months or even a whole year of school. Today, medication is so effective that after an initial two to five day period of treatment, children may attend school without harm to themselves or others. Treatment usually continues for at least a year. Children who are treated with INH because of a positive skin tests and no other symptoms need not miss a single day of school.

PLEURISY

Pleurisy, an infection of the thin outer skin of the lungs, can occur as an infrequent complication of pneumonia or tuberculosis. Pleurisy causes more severe chest pain, higher fever, and occasionally an outpouring of fluid between the lung and the chest wall called *pleural effusion*. Intensive treatment is required.

Pleurisy caused by some of the other viruses can also be present independent of pneumonia. This type of pleurisy almost never causes effusion, although it can cause a moderately severe, constricting type of pain in the chest. Therefore, it has come to be known as the grippe or devil's grippe. It is self-limiting, going away in seven to fourteen days, and requires no antibiotic treatment.

SECTION 6

DISEASES OF THE HEART

Acquired Heart Disease
- Nature of the Condition
- Symptoms and Diagnosis
- School Relevance and Treatment

Rheumatic Fever
- Nature of the Condition
- Symptoms
- School Relevance

Congenital Heart Disease
- Nature of the Condition
- Symptoms
  —Cyanotic Type
  —Noncyanotic Type
- Treatment
- School Relevance
- Role of the School Nurse

Heart Murmurs

ACQUIRED HEART DISEASE

Nature of the Condition

Acquired heart disease can occur in children of school age. It may be caused by viruses, bacteria, or, rarely, fungi, and it can attack a perfectly healthy child. It may occur by itself, but most often it occurs as a complication of another primary disease. This primary disease may be serious, such as diphtheria, or it may be only a mild viral infection.

The heart has three distinct layers: outer, middle, and inner. Infection of the outer layer, or pericardium, is called *pericarditis*. In the middle, or myocardium, it is called *myocarditis;* in the inner layer, or endocardium, it is called *endocarditis.*

Symptoms and Diagnosis

All acquired heart disease makes children seriously ill with fever and prostration. They rarely want to get out of bed. The heart rate is usually quite rapid, even faster than one sees with the same amount of fever from other disease. The heart may also beat irregularly.

School Relevance and Treatment

All acquired heart disease of acute onset as described above makes children so sick that it is unlikely they will be in school. However, if a child appears sicker than the degree of fever would indicate, especially if the heart rate is very rapid and/or irregular, he or she should be allowed to rest in the clinic until the parents can pick him or her up. Definitive treatment will depend on the exact diagnosis and must always be carried out by the child's physician.

RHEUMATIC FEVER

Nature of the Condition

Rheumatic fever is a special type of acquired heart disease that is caused by a particular body sensitivity to the same streptococcus germ that causes scarlet fever and strep throat. After complete recovery from rheumatic fever, a few children are left with heart valves in a damaged condition. Of the four heart valves, the mitral valve is the one

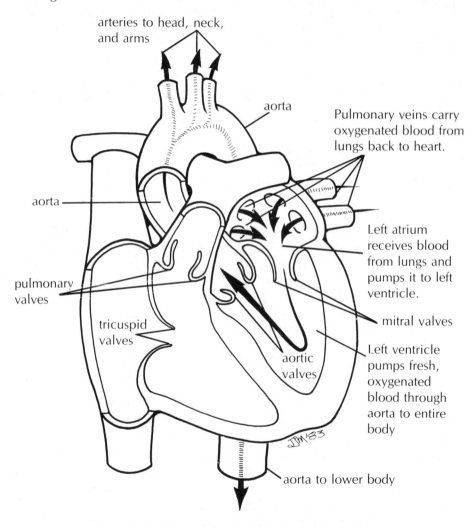

arteries to head, neck, and arms

aorta

Pulmonary veins carry oxygenated blood from lungs back to heart.

aorta

Left atrium receives blood from lungs and pumps it to left ventricle.

pulmonary valves

tricuspid valves

mitral valves

aortic valves

Left ventricle pumps fresh, oxygenated blood through aorta to entire body

aorta to lower body

Figure 6–1. Normal Arterial Circulation in the Heart

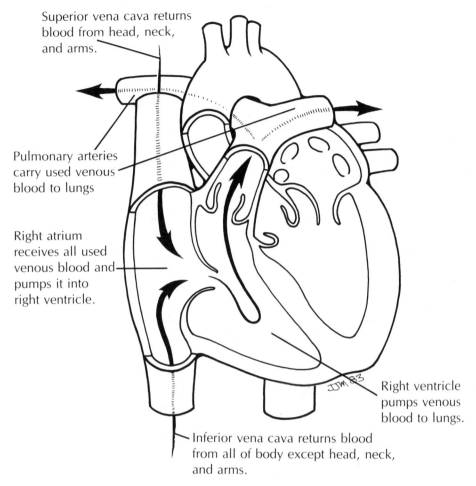

Superior vena cava returns blood from head, neck, and arms.

Pulmonary arteries carry used venous blood to lungs

Right atrium receives all used venous blood and pumps it into right ventricle.

Right ventricle pumps venous blood to lungs.

Inferior vena cava returns blood from all of body except head, neck, and arms.

Figure 6–2. Normal Venous Circulation in the Heart

most commonly involved. After several years, this valvular damage causes symptoms that can gradually become severe.

Symptoms

The early symptoms of chronic rheumatic heart disease are mild shortness of breath, especially on exertion, occasional mild chest pain, and occasionally slight blue color around the lips. Eventually, the heart enlarges a great deal, it weakens, and actual heart failure ensues. It takes several years after the initial attack for significant valvular damage to occur. While most cases of valvular disease do not cause noticeable symptoms until young adult life, occasionally symptoms appear in children of secondary school age.

School Relevance

Some children with chronic rheumatic carditis may be in school. If so, they may have a note from their doctor asking for some restriction of physical activity. If this should occur, the teacher should accede to the doctor's request.

Rheumatic fever is a rare disease, especially in southern climates with milder winters. Recently more cases have been reported in Florida, Arizona, and Utah. School nurses should be alert to this possibility. Better treatment of early streptococcus infections has brought a welcome decline in the incidence of rheumatic heart disease.

CONGENITAL HEART DISEASE

Nature of the Condition

Congenital heart disease is present when the child is born and can be inherited or caused by disease or distress of the embryo during its development. It is usually characterized by a hole between the right and left sides of the heart, an abnormal number of heart chambers, abnormalities of the heart valves or major blood vessels near the heart, abnormal placement or twisting of the heart, or many other variations from normal. There are two types:

1. *Cyanotic.* Arterial blood has a high oxygen content and is bright red; venous blood is dark red because it has a lower oxygen content. As dark red venous blood passes through the lungs, it is reoxygenated and pumped out through the arteries to the body. In most cases of cyanotic congenital heart disease, venous blood escapes through an abnormal opening in the heart, enters into, mixes with, and darkens the arterial blood. This causes cyanosis, a purplish-blue coloration especially visible through the fingernails and in the lips.

2. *Noncyanotic.* When arterial blood is abnormally routed into the venous side of the heart, the mixture goes through the lungs to become oxygenated again before going back out to the body, so it becomes bright red again and the skin color is normal.

Symptoms

Cyanotic Type

1. Cyanotic children exhibit a bluish tinge around the lips and fingertips. After several years the fingertips become swollen. This is called *clubbing.*
2. All of the tissues receive a poor oxygen supply, impairing body growth. Resistance to infection is low; the child is sickly and frequently absent from school.
3. Breathing is deeper and faster to get sufficient oxygen. Very little exercise is tolerated, requiring frequent rest. Chronic shortness of breath makes speaking difficult.
4. The brain receives less oxygen, which impairs cerebral processes in many subtle ways. Many of these children have learning problems.

The extent of the symptoms depends on the amount of the oxygen deficit. Other factors that influence the severity of the symptoms are the size of the heart, the regularity of the heartbeat, and the blood pressure.

Noncyanotic Type

In many cases noncyanotic heart disease causes no symptoms at all, at least in childhood. As the child grows older, the heart gets abnormally large because of the extra workload, having to pump a larger-than-normal volume of blood. The enlarged heart is a weak heart and eventually decompensates (fails). When this happens, the child begins to show many of the same symptoms as the child with cyanotic heart disease.

Treatment

In both types of heart disease in children of school age—cyanotic and noncyanotic—treatment consists of surgical repair of the abnormality. Not all congenital cardiac abnormalities can be repaired. Some are so severe and complicated that complete cure by surgery is impossible. In these cases, palliative procedures often can be performed that give partial relief. In most cases, however, surgical cure is possible.

The modern-day diagnosis and surgical correction of congenital heart disease are complicated and should be done only by a pediatric cardiologist and skilled cardiac surgeon. If their services are not available locally, the child should be taken to a larger medical center.

School Relevance

Many children with congenital heart disease attend school every day. Most are in mainstream regular classes. Some have had operations to correct their heart defects, and some have not.

Children who visit a doctor for regular checkups are fortunate because this type of heart problem is usually diagnosed with a stethoscope. A murmur, by its sound and location, can guide the cardiologist to perform the kinds of tests that lead to an exact diagnosis. There are many children, however, especially in the so-called inner-city schools, who rarely if ever visit a doctor. They may go for years with their hearts slowly enlarging and gradually becoming more and more damaged. By the time they start having symptoms, it is usually too late to effect a complete cure.

Role of the School Nurse

Most children with congenital heart disease will be under a physician's care. The school nurse should maintain contact with the doctor's office for any special instructions that may be necessary. The nurse should also act as an intermediary between the educational and medical personnel to make sure the efforts of both are coordinated for the child's welfare. This will be especially true in these instances:

1. *Special education.* If the child is not performing at academic potential, this may be because of general weakness or lack of oxygen to the brain. The school nurse may contribute to the development of an individual educational plan by pointing out that the child is eligible for special education under the physically handicapped (or "Other Health Impaired") category.

2. *Restriction of physical activity.* Almost all children with congenital heart disease can be allowed to regulate their own activity; they will stop when tired. However, the school nurse may need to reinforce teachers' efforts to keep some overeager children from exceeding their capabilities.

3. *School attendance.* Some principals and teachers are overly fearful when children with symptomatic or cyanotic congenital heart disease attend school. As long as contact can be maintained between doctor, parent or relative, and the school nurse or principal, the child should be encouraged to attend classes as much as possible. Children who have inoperable conditions and a short life span need as much normal activity as they can comfortably tolerate.

HEART MURMURS

Most children with congenital heart disease will have significant murmurs that can be heard with a stethoscope by a physician or by a school nurse with proper training and experience. However, caution is necessary.

Many children have soft, quiet heart murmurs that are called functional. These murmurs are very common—about 50 percent of children have them. They come and go from day to day. *They have absolutely no significance whatsoever. They are normal.*

Functional murmurs are often heard in school screening programs. If proper rechecking is not done, these children, who need not and should not go to a doctor at all, are referred to a doctor. Some of them are subjected to a great many unnecessary tests, some of which may be risky in and of themselves. Furthermore, the children come to think of themselves as having an abnormal heart and develop an unhealthy attitude toward their own physical capabilities.

A pediatric cardiologist can sort out some of these murmurs simply by listening to them, thus sparing the child any tests at all, even a simple x-ray of the chest. Most of the time, only a chest x-ray and electrocardiogram will be necessary—both entirely harmless and painless. Only about 10 to 15 percent of cases referred to most specialists will require invasive techniques (intravenous dye injection or inserting a long flexible tube through a vein into the heart), and this number is gradually getting smaller as a result of the development of new techniques. These latter tests require hospitalization and carry some small risk, though in the presence of serious congenital heart disease they are invaluable and necessary.

DISEASES OF THE BRAIN

Epilepsy
- Nature of the Condition
- Symptoms and School Relevance
  —Grand Mal Seizures
  —Petit Mal Seizures
  —Psychomotor Epilepsy
  —Epileptic Equivalents
- Diagnosis
- Medication for Long-Term Control
  —Prevention of Tongue Biting
- Athletic Participation
- Treatment
  —Emergency On-Site Treatment

Rabies
- Nature of the Condition
- Exposure and School Relevance
- Treatment
  —Management of Biting Animal
  —Management of the Bite
  —Rabies Vaccine

Cerebral Palsy
- Nature of the Condition
- Symptoms
- Classification

- School Relevance
- Treatment
- Role of the School Nurse

Developmental Dyspraxia

Progressive Diseases of the Nervous System
- Nature of the Condition
- Symptoms
- School Relevance and Role of the School Nurse
- Treatment

EPILEPSY

Nature of the Condition

Epilepsy is one of the medical conditions that almost every teacher and school nurse will have to deal with several times during a school career. It is a relatively common affliction and is seen much more often in children than adults. For unknown reasons, most children outgrow their epilepsy during their teens. Also, treatment is effective in most

CLASSIFICATIONS OF SEIZURES

ILAE classification	Other terminology
I. Partial seizures	
A. Simple partial seizures	
1. With motor signs	Jacksonian seizures or focal motor seizures
2. With somatosensory or special sensory (visual, auditory, olfactory, gustatory, vertiginous) symptoms	Sensory seizures
3. With autonomic symptoms or signs	Abdominal epilepsy or epileptic equivalent
B. Complex partial seizures	Psychomotor or temporal lobe seizures
II. Generalized seizures	
A. Absence seizures	
1. Typical	Petit mal
2. Atypical	Petit mal variant or complex petit mal
B. Myoclonic seizures	Myoclonic seizures
C. Atonic seizures	Akinetic seizures or drop attacks
D. Tonic-clonic seizures	Grand mal major motor seizures, generalized convulsive seizures

Commission on Classification and Terminology of the International League Against Epilepsy: Proposal for revised clinical and electroencephalographic classification of epileptic seizures. Epilepsia 22:489, 1981.

cases, and this too can shorten the natural course of a disease which, untreated, can have serious potential.

Each individual epileptic attack or seizure is frightening to school personnel, especially the typical grand mal seizure or major convulsion. However, children are unlikely to harm themselves during a seizure. The major cause of concern is brain damage from repeated, uncontrolled convulsions. During a convulsion, the patient stops breathing for a brief period of time and the entire body is deprived of oxygen. The brain—the organ most sensitive to lack of oxygen—suffers most, and a number of brain cells die when the brain is deprived of oxygen. Once a brain cell dies it never regenerates, and eventually, with the death of enough cells, learning disability or mental retardation may result. It is well known that many kinds of brain damage are more common in epileptics.

Most epileptics are normal in all respects aside from their occasional seizures. Those who have severe and frequent attacks, however, either because of poor compliance with medical treatment or because their disease is so severe, often develop some degree of noticeable brain damage. Also, since pathology in one part of the brain is often associated with abnormalities in other parts, even well-controlled epileptics have a higher incidence of subtle learning and behavior problems as well as a higher incidence of frank intellectual retardation.

Symptoms and School Relevance

Epilepsy is often classified by the nature of the seizure, and different types often respond best to different medications. There are many types of seizures, but only four will be discussed here. The others are rare or only seen in infancy.

Grand Mal Seizures

Tonic phase. This is a typical hard-shaking convulsion. It is liable to occur at any time, but some authorities feel it is more likely to occur when the child is at rest than when engaged in some sort of mental or physical activity. It sometimes begins with an aura—seeing a light or halo, or having an unusual feeling. At this time, the child is still conscious and will appear frightened. Almost immediately, however, the convulsion will begin with a sudden, rigid stiffening of the entire body—so stiff and so strong that the back is arched, and if the child were able to be balanced on his back, the heels and head would touch the ground. The instant this begins, consciousness is lost and the child falls to the ground. This is called the *tonic* phase of the convulsion, during which all of the muscles of the body are held extremely tightly. The jaw is tightly clenched and no effort should be made to open it. Broken teeth (and lawsuits) have resulted from overzealous efforts.

Clonic Phase. After about twenty to forty seconds the *clonic* phase begins. During this second phase, the true shaking convulsion begins because of intermittent contractions of body muscles. It is during this period that one may safely insert a padded stick between the teeth provided it is done slowly and gently.

The third stage is one of deep sleep and lasts five to thirty minutes. Following this stage, the child awakens and, except for muscle soreness, is as normal as before.

What has been described here is a typical or average convulsion, though any one convulsion or one of its phases is apt to be a little bit different—longer or shorter, more or less severe. Sometimes, in a mild attack, there is no period of deep sleep. Sometimes the seizure is limited to one side of the body or only one extremity with no loss of consciousness. These are called *Jacksonian seizures.*

Petit Mal Seizures

Petit mal seizures are also called *absence spells.* They are brief episodes, lasting one to three seconds, during which the child loses consciousness but does not lose body tone and usually does not fall down. If the child is holding something—a pencil or glass—he or she is apt to drop it. During this brief period the child is completely out of contact. When the episode is over, the child will resume activity, completely unaware that anything has happened.

The child with petit mal epilepsy often has twenty to forty episodes a day. As with grand mal seizures, there usually are some variations in the appearance of the seizures. There may be occasional twitching of the facial or arm muscles. Sometimes an attack can last five to ten seconds. Many are so brief that nobody ever knows they have occurred. Contrary to grand mal seizures, this type of epilepsy is not associated with brain damage.

Teachers often wonder if certain children have petit mal epilepsy because they lack attention or stare out of the window or do not hear something that was said, and they will refer the child to a physician.

Many doctors have been upset about this because, even though they feel sure from the described symptoms that the child does not have epilepsy, once the suspicion has been raised they are obligated to proceed with some fairly expensive tests (EEG, x-ray, etc.), which most of the time show normal results. However, classroom experience shows that teachers do have some reason to wonder about some children.

It is difficult to give good guidelines about which episodes may be petit mal attacks and which are simply wandering attention. One important factor is frequency of occurrence. If the spell only occurs occasionally, not even every day, it is more likely to be just lack of attention. Also, if the teacher looks closely, the pupils of the eyes will always be enlarged during a petit mal seizure and they will not constrict even if a bright light is shined into them. If the child is touched during an episode, he or she will not notice it. If the child drops whatever he or she may be holding, this is also suggestive evidence.

In summary, if the teacher or school nurse is not sure and if the attacks are infrequent, it is better to wait and watch until more definitive signs appear. This course of action will result in less anxiety and less needless expense for the family.

Psychomotor Epilepsy

Psychomotor epilepsy is a rare type of epilepsy in which an attack causes the patient to engage suddenly in a spurt of coordinated muscular activity that may appear to be under voluntary control.

The seizures are characteristically of brief duration, lasting from a minute to 5 to 10 minutes. Consciousness is often impaired but rarely completely lost. The most common motor symptoms are drawing or jerking of the mouth and face . . . Aphasia or dysphasia may be present . . . The eyes may stare in a searching manner. There may be tonic posturing or a desire to urinate. Coordinated but inappropriate movements may be performed repeatedly in a stereotyped manner (automatism), common examples being clutching, fumbling, kicking, walking or running in circles, swallowing, smacking, chewing, licking, and spitting. Pill-rolling, . . . [twisting hand or arm movements,] or flinging movements [of the arms] are less common. Inhibitory seizures with loss of tone (limpness) or arrest of motion (freezing) may occur. Affective expressions such as laughing or crying are not unusual. . . . When the attack is over, there may or may not be . . . sluggishness or sleep. Amnesia of the attack is the rule. (From Barnett, *Pediatrics*, 15th Ed. used with permission from Appleton-Century-Crofts.)

Epileptic Equivalents

Episodic vomiting, diarrhea, dizziness, vertigo, and even episodes of seeming insanity have been blamed on epilepsy. Needless to say, these common symptoms are rarely caused by epilepsy. A pediatrician can easily rule out epilepsy in more than 99 percent of cases of this nature. Diagnosis of that one remaining percent is difficult even for skillful neurologists using all of the diagnostic tools at their command.

Diagnosis

Certain factors are common to all forms of epilepsy:

1. *Sudden onset and relatively rapid termination.* Epilepsy usually begins when least expected, for no apparent reason, runs its course, and stops.

2. *Loss of memory.* Memory loss occurs in all forms of epilepsy except the epileptic equivalents. Remembrance of the episode is so unusual in epilepsy that it makes some neurologists skeptical that there is actually a condition called epileptic equivalents. Typically, when epileptic attacks are over, patients awaken in a dazed state wondering what happened to them. If they have suffered many attacks, they will be able to guess what happened but will not remember it.

3. *Repeated attacks.* It is very rare for a person with epilepsy to have a single attack. Occasionally a child will be diagnosed and treated after the first attack and never have another, but this is quite rare.

When all three of the above factors are present, the diagnosis is easier to make. Physicians, however, will want to confirm the diagnosis with various laboratory tests. Those commonly ordered are an electro-encephalogram (brain wave test) and x-rays of the head. In fairly typical cases, these two tests are all that are necessary. More extensive computerized x-rays, blood tests, dye injections, spinal taps, and other tests may be required in complicated cases.

Figure 7–1 will help distinguish between real and pseudo seizures.

DIFFERENTIAL DIAGNOSIS BETWEEN REAL AND PSEUDO SEIZURES

A. *SYNCOPE* (simple fainting)
1. Situational (e.g., standing, after voiding, or brushing hair)
2. In adolescence or preadolescence
3. No trismus or incontinence
4. May have a few jerking movements
5. EEG usually normal

GRAND MAL (TONIC-CLONIC)
1. Not dependant on situation (but may be associated with lack of sleep or food)
2. At any age
3. May have trismus or incontinence
4. Jerking movements are prominent
5. EEG usually abnormal

B. *DAYDREAMING*
1. Lasts minutes
2. Eyelids don't flutter
3. EEG normal

PETIT MAL (ABSENCE)
1. Lasts seconds
2. Eyelids flutter
3. EEG definitely abnormal

C. *AGGRESSIVE OR BIZARRE BEHAVIOR*
1. No definite beginning or end
2. Doesn't end in grand mal
3. No aura or vague aura
4. Is influenced by environment
5. EEG usually normal

PSYCHOMOTOR SEIZURES
1. Clear difference between seizure and nonseizure state
2. May conclude with grand mal
3. Aura is clear and repetitive
4. Is usually independent of environment
5. EEG usually abnormal, especially in sleep (24-hour trace may be necessary)

D. *PSEUDO OR HYSTERICAL SEIZURES*
1. Influenced by environment
2. Serves a psychological role (e.g., attention getting)
3. Patient will not ordinarily hurt self
4. EEG usually normal even during seizure

REAL SEIZURES (GRAND MAL)
1. Independent of environment
2. Serves no psychological role
3. Patient may inadvertently hurt self
4. EEG usually abnormal

Figure 7–1.

Medication for Long-Term Control

Epilepsy can be both the easiest and the most difficult of all diseases to treat. It is extremely capricious. Some cases will respond well to a single harmless medication. Other cases require as many as three or four types of medicine, all given several times a day. In these difficult cases, the medicines themselves usually cause some unpleasant side effects and the attending physician must monitor the child frequently.

Recently, epilepsy specialists have been emphasizing the importance of giving as few drugs as possible. This is laudable. If a school nurse encounters a child on more than two or three medications at a time, the school consultant physician should be advised.

The medicine must be continued for at least two to five years. Some neurologists have a standing rule that medications must be given for four years after the last convulsion or seizure. If treatment is stopped too soon, the attacks may return with greater severity. For this reason, some feel it is better not to begin treatment after the first attack. Some physicians follow this policy, reasoning that one seizure does not cause ill effects and it may be possible to save the patient four years of drug therapy and emotional trauma. Some children have one typical grand mal seizure and never have another.

All forms of epilepsy are treated by oral medication. The schedule can usually be arranged so the child need not take any doses during school hours. This is by far the best arrangement. If the physician has sound medical reasons for requiring the child to take a dose during school hours, the school authorities should cooperate. However, the psychological effects on the child are so important that the school nurse, principal, or counselor should have a conference with the parent and explore the possibility of giving all doses at home.

Prevention of Tongue Biting

For many years, doctors advised the insertion of a padded tongue blade or other object between the teeth during a grand mal convulsion. This was meant to prevent a person from seriously biting the tongue during a clonic convulsion. Instead, it caused broken teeth and cuts and bruises of the lips and mouth. Long-term studies over the past five to seven years have shown that patients do *not* bite their tongue during a convulsion. Therefore, most doctors advise not putting anything between the teeth.

Athletic Participation

Children with well-controlled epilepsy can participate in almost all activities. There are two sports that must be considered dangerous for children with epilepsy: gymnastics (rope climbing, parallel bars, swinging rings, trampolines) and swimming, especially under water. Since some children have a history of seizures on hyperventilation, proper preconditioning is essential.

There is more concern and more controversy over participation in football than in any other sport. A seizure on the playing field would be no more harmful than the same seizure anywhere else, but there is a fear that a head injury might aggravate the preexisting epileptic condition and cause more frequent seizures. Actually, there is no good medical evidence to support this fear. However, the general feeling prevails that a child should be in top physical condition and free of all illness to play this injury-prone sport. A child with epilepsy who is determined, and who is a valuable player besides, will probably find a way to play. If such is the case, it should be only with full knowledge by all concerned of all risks involved. Sometimes a trial period in middle school can be helpful in deciding future plans so that by high school a decision has already been made and agreed upon.

Treatment

Emergency On-Site Treatment

The best treatment for grand mal seizures is to let the child be, let the convulsion run its course, and let the child sleep until he or she awakens. Unfortunately, it is almost impossible to keep somebody from rubbing the chest, loosening the clothing, or something else equally ineffective. The more stimulation the child receives, the longer the seizure is apt to last, so the less touching the better. As the seizure is about to end, it is a good idea to turn the child on the side so that any secretions or vomitus will run out of the mouth and not back down the throat.

It is an often-stated medical dictum that patients never die during a convulsion. There is a condition, however, called *status epilepticus*, in which the seizure continues for fifteen to thirty minutes or longer. Even in these cases the patient does not die, but there is greater danger of brain damage. The dilemma that often arises is, how long is too long? After what length of time should the child be taken to the nearest hospital emergency room or doctor's office? If the child is still convulsing after five minutes, he or she should be taken to the nearest medical facility and given the proper medication to stop the seizure promptly. This usually consists of some intravenous medication such as a barbiturate or Valium.

The other types of epilepsy need no emergency treatment except to prevent the child from self harm.

RABIES

Nature of the Condition

Rabies is an infection of the brain (*encephalitis*) caused by a specific virus which can affect many mammals. The most common domestic animals infected are dogs and cats, but horses, cows, and other livestock are susceptible. The largest reservoir is in wild animals, and the animals most commonly affected are skunks, foxes, coyotes, bobcats, raccoons, and bats.

Rodents such as squirrels, hamsters, guinea pigs, gerbils, chipmunks, rats, mice, and rabbits are so rarely infected with rabies that health departments often do not even test these animals when people report that they were bitten, and their bites almost never require antirabies treatment.

Exposure and School Relevance

Most commonly, exposure is caused by an animal bite. A nonbite exposure, however, can come from a scratch, abrasion, or other open wound or sore contaminated with animal saliva. Excluding these, a casual contact such as petting a rabid animal is not considered an exposure. (Airborne exposure, as in a bat cave, is very rare; only two cases have been reported.)

Bats are a frequent cause for concern, but it is extremely rare for a bat to bite. Vampire bats, the only bat that actually bites, are not found in the United States. Frequently at school, children will pick up a dead bat and play with it. These bats should be sent to the local health department for examination. If rabies virus is found in the bat's brain, each child who played with it must be evaluated individually by a physician to determine the need for rabies vaccine.

Treatment

Management of Biting Animal

Because the disease is so horrible and fatal, any suspected exposure must be handled without compromise. Should a child be bitten on the school grounds by a domestic animal, it is important for the animal to be chained or placed in an escape-proof cage and observed for ten days. The incubation period of rabies in an animal is less than two weeks. Therefore, if symptoms do not develop in ten to fourteen days, it is safe to assume the animal is not rabid. If a previously healthy dog or cat develops rabies, one of the first things it often does is run away. Therefore, if a child has been bitten by an animal that cannot be found, it must be assumed that the child has been exposed to rabies, and antirabies vaccine must be given.

If a domestic animal develops symptoms of rabies, it should be humanely killed and the head packed in ice until the brain can be examined for rabies. Previously, it was necessary to wait for the animal to die of rabies before examining the brain. Current techniques enable rabies to be identified in the brain at any stage of the disease.

Nothing is more important than identifying the animal and catching it. The police should be notified immediately. Capture and observation of a domestic animal is better than killing it. No matter how small the chance that the animal was sick, no matter how much pity the parent has for the child needing shots, an alternative is not to be considered. The same is true in deciding whether or not to destroy a much-loved pet. Wild animals should be killed and the heads examined as soon as possible.

Management of the Bite

Immediate and thorough washing of the wound using lots of water is very effective and in all probability prevents some cases of rabies, especially in nonbite exposures.

The child should be referred to a physician as soon as possible. Many decisions must be made, such as what type of antirabies vaccine should be used and which child needs treatment. Modern treatment usually consist of five or six injections, in contrast to the previously required fourteen to twenty-one.

Rabies Vaccine

The original rabies vaccine was made from the spinal cord of rabid monkeys. It was effective but the rate of adverse reactions was high. One of the most serious reactions was a permanent paralysis of the legs and occasionally death from paralysis of the respiratory muscles.

Vaccine grown in duck eggs became available in the mid-1950s. It is more effective in preventing rabies, and the incidence of serious reaction is much lower.

More recently, a vaccine grown in human cells has become available, and so far it has not only proved the most effective in preventing rabies, but serious reactions have not been reported. It is called human diploid cell vaccine or HDCV.

Rabies immune globulin is also available and is usually used in conjunction with HDCV.

CEREBRAL PALSY

Nature of the Condition

Cerebral palsy is a relatively common disorder seen in schools. It is caused by disease of the brain itself. In most cases, the brain is damaged by disease or injury during fetal life, during the birth process, or shortly after birth.

The nervous system includes the brain, spinal cord, and peripheral nerves. Nerves originate in the brain, go down the spinal cord, and then diverge throughout the body. If a nerve is damaged in the brain or spinal cord, the muscle it supplies becomes fixed in spasm. If that same nerve is damaged after emerging from the spinal cord, the muscle it supplies becomes paralyzed in flaccidity. (Diseases of the peripheral nerves, such as poliomyelitis, produce a flaccid paralysis.)

Since the primary damage is in the brain, the muscles controlled by that part of the brain are paralyzed but they are fixed in spasm and the child is said to have a spastic paralysis. For this reason, many victims of cerebral palsy are referred to as *spastics*.

Cerebral palsy results from damage to the motor areas, the parts of the brain that send messages out to the muscles—not the part of the brain that receives messages through the sense organs. This concept is basic to an understanding of the difficult life of many of these victims, at least half of whom have good intelligence and an understanding of everything that is going on around them but no way of communicating that understanding.

Symptoms

The nerves that control the muscles of speech, facial expression, and coordinated and controlled arm and leg movement, and those that hold the body in an upright position, all originate in the motor areas of the brain. These nerves are damaged at their very point of origin, and messages transmitted are garbled in severe and bizarre ways. A child who wants to smile may grimace; if the child tries to cry, he or she may smile or laugh or emit weird sounds. Drooling is frequent. The child may be completely unable to speak or be completely unintelligible.

Arm, leg, and trunk muscle involvement causes limping, shuffling gait, unwanted and uncoordinated movements, and falling to the ground.

Generalized convulsions are common, as are convulsions of individual arms or legs or both.

General intelligence or IQ varies considerably; some children are of average or superior intelligence, while others are severely retarded. Testing is often very difficult and frequently requires special skills and special tests.

Classification

1. *Hemiplegia.* Only one side of the body is involved. The arm is usually less useful than the leg, though the child almost always walks with some limp. This is the most common form.

2. *Monoplegia.* Rarely, only one extremity is involved. In most cases, involvement of the other extremity on the same side can be demonstrated with stress tests.

3. *Quadriplegia.* All four extremities are involved, but usually the legs are worse than the arms.

4. *Paraplegia.* Only the legs are involved.

5. *Diplegia.* All four extremities are involved, with very little noticeable arm involvement.

6. *Athetosis.* This produces unwanted and uncontrollable bizarre body, extremity, and/or facial movements.

7. *Dystonia.* Uncontrollable body muscle tone results in abnormal body postures.

8. *Ataxia.* The child has difficulty or inability in sitting or standing upright, or moving without holding on.

9. *Atonia.* The child is very limp with no muscle tone. This is rare and mainly seen in infants.

10. *Mixed.* This form includes various mixtures of the above.

School Relevance

Many children with cerebral palsy can attend regular classes. They will obviously need some help, both academically and physically.

Cerebral palsy can be so severe as to preclude standing, walking, or learning any self-help skills such as feeding or using the toilet. On the other hand, the condition can be so mild that the child is just thought to be excessively clumsy. In these latter cases, the true diagnosis may not be made for many years. Indeed, neurologists sometimes disagree on whether or not a particular child has cerebral palsy.

Treatment

There are five basic forms of treatment:

1. *Medications* are used primarily to control convulsions. All of the various medications used in epilepsy are available. Sometimes, medication will be used to control spasm.

2. *Surgery* is used to lengthen short muscles or tendons and to reinsert tendons into different locations to increase utility of the arms or legs. Many other surgical procedures are beneficial.

3. *Physiotherapy* is useful in almost all cases of cerebral palsy. The earlier it is started, the better the results, and it should be in place long before children start school.

4. *Occupational therapy* helps children learn the skills of daily living, such as sitting, feeding, and writing. This should begin as early as physiotherapy.

5. *Counseling* is necessary for parents as well as children. Both have great need for psychological support and help in a school situation. Counselors who are themselves handicapped often make excellent therapists.

Role of the School Nurse

Obviously, in very mild cases the school nurse will need do no more than for the regular school child. However, most cases will require special nursing knowledge and procedures.

1. *Charting.* Extra care will be required for medication, physiotherapy, and other nursing procedures. The school nurse should keep a chart somewhat similar to a hospital chart that will provide a daily or weekly log.

2. *Medication.* A large proportion of children with cerebral palsy receive medication; many have difficulty swallowing. The school nurse should give the medication and record each dose. The nurse also needs to be aware of adverse reactions to the medicines; a current copy of the PDR (*Physician's Desk Reference*) should be available.

3. *Coordination of physiotherapy and occupational therapy at home and at school.* In many cases therapy is given only at the school or only at the medical office. The school nurse can be instrumental in coordination of services.

4. *Counseling.* In cooperation with the school guidance counselor, the nurse can help the parent accept the child's condition and not continue to seek miracle cures. At the same time, parents must be encouraged to continue therapies that are known to be beneficial.

DEVELOPMENTAL DYSPRAXIA

This is a relatively rare neurological disorder that is also called the *clumsy child syndrome*. All school nurses and teachers will see these children during their careers. The brain pathology is different from that of cerebral palsy, but there is an obvious problem with muscular coordination in this condition also. These children are more than a little clumsy, and they also have a higher than normal incidence of learning problems.

Children who are mentally retarded may also be clumsy. The dyspraxic child is assumed to have normal general intelligence, even though he or she may perform poorly in school. These children will have their greatest problems as they approach ten to twelve years of age, as this is when normal children begin to become quite skillful in athletics. Physical education teachers need to be especially alert to such children because they will need a great deal of encouragement and special tasks commensurate with their ability. Some of the common characteristics of this condition include an awkward and shambling gait, frequent falls when running, poor dressing ability, spilling milk, messy eating, poor handwriting, slow reaction time, and poor ability in almost any type of organized or competitive sport.

PROGRESSIVE DISEASES OF THE NERVOUS SYSTEM

Nature of the Condition

The word *progressive* indicates an ongoing disease process during which the symptoms get worse. Examples of such diseases are multiple sclerosis, brain tumor, and encephalitis. Physicians frequently refer to this group of diseases as progressive central nervous system disease.

Symptoms

The specific symptoms of progressive disease vary greatly. For example, encephalitis or meningitis can cause a child to become severely ill overnight, whereas brain tumors or multiple sclerosis usually progress slowly. In all cases, however, the disease becomes steadily worse, albeit sometimes very slowly.

School Relevance and Role of the School Nurse

There are certain conditions in which the earliest symptoms that can be seen are subtle changes in the higher cognitive functions such as short-term memory, arithmetic ability, or abstract reasoning. If the motor area of the brain is involved, a change in writing or athletic ability may be noticed.

Since progressive nervous system disease of subtle onset is quite rare, caution should be exercised in notifying parents about such symptoms. However, if a change from previous abilities or a noticeable change in behavior occurs, it would be well for the school nurse to speak with the parent. This may lead to an early diagnosis and thus render the disease a bit more amenable to treatment.

Treatment

Progressive disease is always treated by a physician; the specific treatment is always dependent on the diagnosis.

DISEASES WITH SPECIAL SCHOOL RELEVANCE

Acquired Immune Deficiency Syndrome (AIDS)
- Nature of the disorder
- Congenital AIDS
- Risk Factors
- Prevention and Treatment
- AIDS Education
- School Relevance
- Role of the School Nurse

Infectious Mononucleosis (IM)
- School Relevance
- Symptoms and Diagnosis
- Complications
- Treatment
  —Chronic Infectious Mononucleosis

Viral Hepatitis
- Nature of the Condition
- Varieties
  —Hepatitis A
  —Hepatitis B
  —Laboratory Differentiation of Hepatitis A and B
- Treatment

- Prevention of Hepatitis A
  - —Handwashing
  - —Gamma Globulin (GG)
- Prevention of Hepatitis B
- School Relevance
  - —How Frequent and How Dangerous Is Hepatitis
  - —Cleaning of Classrooms
  - —Reporting to Parents and Health Department
  - —Who Gets Immune Globulin?

Reye Syndrome

- Symptoms
- Differential Diagnosis
- Pathology
- Relationship to Aspirin
- School Relevance

Venereal Disease

- Sex Education
- School Relevance
- Relating to Health Department
- Routes of Transmission

Syphilis

- Nature of the Condition
- Symptoms and Stages
  - —Primary
  - —Secondary
  - —Tertiary
- Treatment

Gonorrhea

- Nature of the condition
- Symptoms
- Treatment

Nonspecific Urethritis and Other Genital Infections

- Nature of the Condition
- Symptoms
- Treatment

Other Venereal Diseases

- Nature of the Condition

ACQUIRED IMMUNE DEFICIENCY SYNDROME (AIDS)

AIDS was first reported in the U.S. in 1981. It was probably imported from Africa where it had been causing disease in humans for many years. Where was the disease before Africans began to have it?

The present theory is that it has long existed as a virus in monkeys, although it did not cause them symptoms of illness. The virus then mutated and became capable of infecting humans and in its mutated form attacked the human T-cell lymphocytes—the cells responsible for providing immunity to infection. This slow destruction of natural body immunity causes the chain of events leading to the three stages of the disease.

Since 1981 AIDS has been spreading rapidly. It exists in all age groups and both sexes, but because of the usual methods of transmission it is more prevalent in males. The following chart represents the dramatic increase in reported cases in the U.S. between 1981 and 1988. As of March 21, 1988 54,233 cases had been reported in the U.S. (*MMWR*, May 13, 1988)

Year	No. of Cases	Fatality Rate
1981	271	92%
1982	1014	88%
1983	2824	87%
1984	5700	81%
1985	10,109	75%
1986	15,088	54%
1987	15,184	27%

The AIDS virus belongs to a family called the retroviruses. These viruses are capable of reversing the normal RNA-DNA sequence, hence "retro." The virus can be found in all body fluids but primarily in the blood, since that is where most lymphocytes are. It is also found in vaginal secretions and semen in moderate amounts. The amount in saliva, urine, stool, stomach content, and tears is smaller.

AIDS is found mostly in male homosexuals, intravenous drug abusers, prostitutes, and hemophiliacs. Newborn children of mothers with AIDS often develop congenital AIDS, a condition which may be seen in school children. Because of its blood-borne nature, and because anal intercourse often tears the rectum and causes bleeding, males or females who engage in this practice are at high risk. Prostitutes, male and female, are also at high risk because they have sexual contact with so many different individuals. Intravenous drug abusers often share unsterilized needles, causing direct blood-to-blood transmission. Since many prostitutes are intravenous drug abusers, they are doubly at risk. Hemophiliacs require frequent blood transfusions. Any child who received frequent blood transfusions between 1978 and 1985 is at risk. In 1986 the incidence of AIDS in hemophiliacs was about sixteen per 1,000. Blood used for transfusions is now screened, greatly reducing the chance of an individual contracting AIDS by transfusion. It is estimated there is a one in 40,000 chance of acquiring AIDS in this manner.

Nature of the Disorder

The AIDS virus has had at least three names: Human T-cell Lymphocyte Virus, Strain III; (HTLV-III); Lymphadenopathy Virus (LAV); and Human Immunodeficiency Virus (HIV). HIV is now the official name, and everybody hopes it will not be necessary to change it again.

Stage I. When HIV first invades the body, it calls forth a normal antibody response. There is a simple blood test that detects this antibody, and persons with a positive test are called HIV carriers. They are completely asymptomatic, but presumably they can transmit the disease and can themselves later develop AIDS.

Stage II. After a period of two to four years, about 5 to 20 percent of persons who are HIV positive go on to develop Aids Related Complex (ARC), a disease with distinct symptoms: low grade fever, enlarged lymph nodes, night sweats, fatigue, weakness, weight loss, and in some cases, skin and mouth rashes.

Stage III. After one to three years, about 20 to 25 percent of persons with ARC develop AIDS. To be officially classified with AIDS, a patient must exhibit one of a list of "opportunistic infections"—diseases caused by germs, viruses, or fungi that are widely prevalent, but normal immunity prevents the disease from invading the body. These germs are all resistant to antibiotics, so when they invade a person with no immunity, the disease progresses unchecked and is usually fatal. So far, AIDS is a fatal disease, but newer medicines are constantly being tried.

Congenital Aids

Women with AIDS who become pregnant are likely to pass the disease to their fetus during pregnancy. The newborn baby is then actually born with AIDS, and symptoms develop in the first year of life.

The most notable finding is brain damage. It appears that the HIV actually attacks the brain cells in addition to the T-cell lymphocytes, thus causing an encephalitis. The children also develop the opportunistic infections if they live long enough.

Congenital AIDS is fatal, but some children may live long enough to attend school. The same policies that apply to any other child with AIDS would be followed.

Risk Factors

- *Intravenous drug abusers*—from sharing unsterilized needles.
- *Sexual promiscuity.* People who have had only one sexual partner for the past ten years (who do not fall in other risk categories) are at no risk.
- *Anal intercourse*—because of anal bleeding and increased susceptibility of the cells lining the inside of the rectum.
- *Contact with prostitutes* of either sex.
- *Oral sex.*
- *Vaginal intercourse* between a bisexual male and his heterosexual spouse.
- Receiving *blood transfusions* is low risk now that blood is tested. (Donating blood cannot give AIDS.)

Prevention and Treatment

Prevention consists of avoiding all the risk factors. In addition, males should always wear a condom if there is any possibility that a partner has been exposed or if he himself could transmit AIDS.

Treatment during the HIV positive and ARC stages consists of preventing any further exposure to the virus. In addition, good nutrition, exercise, adequate rest, and other healthful habits are encouraged.

There are medications used to treat the opportunistic infections that occur during Stage-III AIDS. Recent evidence suggests they may actually slow the growth of the virus itself. They are beneficial in that they slow the course of the disease.

AIDS Education

Explicit sex education, beginning at the latest in the sixth grade, is being encouraged by the U.S. Surgeon General. He recommends teaching about promiscuity, homosexuality and heterosexuality, and condoms. Such specificity will be new and frightening to most school districts, and it remains to be seen how much his recommendations will be followed.

Since this call for a massive program of AIDS education in the nation's schools, many states' educational and medical organizations have developed guidelines and curricula for use in student and staff education. Following is a partial list and where they may be obtained:

- *Acquired Immunodeficiency Syndrome (AIDS Secondary Level Curriculum Resources Packet)*, Connecticut Departments of Education and Health Services, Hartford, CT (April 1987)

- *AIDS Instructional Guide for Teachers Grades K–12*, c/o Deputy Commissioner for Elementary, Secondary, and Continuing Education, State Education Department, University of New York, Albany, NY 12234 (1987)

- *Family Living Including Sex Education: Supplementary Material Related to AIDs*, New York City Board of Education, Office of Curriculum Development and Support, Office of the Chancellor, 110 Livingston Street, Brooklyn, NY 11201 (1986)

- *Teacher Curriculum Guide on AIDS*, c/o Elizabeth Stoller, Department of Public Health, Bureau of Disease Control, 101 Grove Street, San Francisco, CA 94102

- *AIDS and Adolescents*, Resources for Educators, Education Department, Center for Population Options, 1012 14th Street, N.W., Washington, D.C. 20005 (July 1987)

- *AIDS Information/Education Plan to Prevent and Control AIDS in the United States,* U.S. Department of Health and Human Services, Public Health Services (March 1987)
- *Report of the Surgeon General's Workshop on Children with HIV Infection and Their Families: Recommendations of Work Group IV,* U.S. Department of Health and Human Services, Public Health Services, DHHS Publication No. HRS-DMC87-1 (March 1987, pages 57–59)
- *Dealing with AIDS—Breaking the Chain of Infection: Guidelines for Schools,* American Association of School Administrators, 1801 N. Moore Street, Arlington, VA 22209 (1988)
- *Guidelines for Effective School Health Education to Prevent the Spread of AIDS,* Morbidity and Mortality Weekly Reports, Centers for Disease Control (January 29, 1988; Vol. 37, No. S-2)

The following have been awarded federal cooperative agreements to develop educational material and curricula.

State Education Agencies: CA, CO, CT, DC, FL, LA, MD, MA, MI, NJ, NY, OH, PA, WA, and PR.

Local Education Agencies: Baltimore City, Boston, Chicago, Miami, Dallas, Denver, Los Angeles, New York City, New Orleans, Philadelphia, San Francisco, and Seattle.

School Relevance

Guidelines have been adopted by most medical and legal authorities which recommend that children with HIV, ARC, and AIDS be allowed to attend school. Most school districts have accepted these guidelines. Since AIDS has never been shown to be spread by airborne or other nonintimate contact, these guidelines seem reasonable.

The following precautions are recommended:

1. Children with AIDS who bite, vomit, have open sores, who drool excessively, or who cannot control their bowels or bladder should be excluded.

2. All body fluids that are spilled (vomit, urine, etc.) by ANY child should be wiped up with a 1 to 10 dilution of chlorox while wearing plastic gloves.

3. Trash cans should have plastic liners.

4. Children with AIDS are more susceptible to infection, so they need to be sent home during outbreaks of usual childhood diseases, such as chicken pox or influenza.

5. The child's privacy should be respected. Only those with a need to know should be told the child has AIDS. This usually includes the principal, counselor, teachers, and school nurse, but may include any person whose duties bring him/her in contact with the student.

6. The risk of contracting AIDS from a child with a nose bleed or minor skin trauma is miniscule. Therefore the following guidelines are suggested.

   a. For caretakers with no open sores on the hands, gloves are optional. Hand washing after caring for the child is sufficient.

   b. For caretakers with open hand sores, gloves should be worn.

   c. In no case, should the care of a bleeding child be delayed because of a lack of gloves.

7. Children excluded from school should be provided with an appropriate alternative education.

Role of the School Nurse

The school nurse should act as the main liaison between the doctor, parent, child, and educational personnel. Many activities need to be coordinated: medications, excused absences, homebound teachers, and calls to the doctor's office.

Educational activities are important. Many questions will come from faculty, and more and more, calls will come from health and science teachers asking the nurse to act as a resource person for classroom teaching of students.

AIDS is still a new and puzzling disease, and as newer information unfolds, more questions will be answered and some old answers will change. The school nurse, by remaining informed about new developments, can be helpful to the entire faculty.

Legal issues are important. Each state has laws governing confidentiality and school attendance for children with contagious diseases. Since September 1987, Texas has had a special law for AIDS. The right of the child to attend school and the right of the school staff to know if a child with AIDS is in attendance are often in conflict. The school nurse can help guide school district policy.

INFECTIOUS MONONUCLEOSIS (IM)

A relatively common disease, infectious mononucleosis (IM) is sometimes called glandular fever or "mono." It is caused by a virus that belongs to the herpes family. It is called the Epstein-Barr virus (EBV).

It is contagious, but only mildly so, and is transferred by hand-to-mouth contact, or more directly by kissing. It is, therefore, also called the "kissing disease." Following recovery, a patient may continue to be intermittently contagious for prolonged periods.

Children living in poor socioeconomic circumstances have a higher incidence of IM, probably because of living closer together and increased physical contact. Also, they usually have milder disease because less virus is transferred by hand-to-mouth contact. Symptoms are often more severe among college students, a selected, more affluent group that develops the disease less frequently and at a later age, probably due to less exposure while young and to transfer of larger amounts of virus due to kissing.

School Relevance

Many seem to regard infectious mononucleosis as a more serious disease than it really is. The mortality rate is extremely low, lower than for measles. The incidence of serious complications (encephalitis and hepatitis) is also quite low. The disease confers a permanent immunity, so second attacks are rare. Apart from its somewhat prolonged course, it is a disease that should occasion no alarm. By the time the child returns to school, he or she should be able to participate fully in most activities and will no longer be contagious.

Symptoms and Diagnosis

Symptoms are:

• high fever
• severe sore throat
• membranous exudate on the tonsils

- enlarged tender lymph nodes in the neck
- lesser enlargement of the lymph nodes in the rest of the body
- enlarged spleen
- in some cases, measles-like rash

Infectious mononucleosis lasts longer than most contagious diseases in children; often, the fever will last ten to fourteen days, and a feeling of weakness and tiredness may persist for several weeks. For this reason, and because the disease may be quite mild in younger children, an incorrect diagnosis is often made in children who have a mild sore throat with low-grade fever that lasts more than six or seven days. Several reliable laboratory tests are now available, many of them highly specific, so errors in diagnosis should be much less common.

Complications

Though rare, the following complications may occur:

- encephalitis
- hepatitis
- ruptured spleen
- facial paralysis
- bleeding under the skin

Treatment

Bed rest is necessary only in severe cases. Children and adolescents may walk around if they feel strong enough but should not participate in athletics or excessive physical activities such as jogging. *Contact sports are especially dangerous* because of possible rupture of a fragile, enlarged spleen. Diet can be unrestricted.

For young adults with severe symptoms, steroids have been helpful in lessening the symptoms, but not in shortening the course of the disease. Penicillins of various kinds have been used because of the membranous tonsillitis. There is no evidence that this treatment is helpful, and it often causes skin rashes (especially ampicillin).

Chronic Infectious Mononucleosis

There are now several authoritative virologists who are convinced that IM can persist in low-grade form for several years. This is referred to as Chronic IM (CIM). It is widely discussed in popular magazines and has been called "raggedy-man syndrome." The symptoms of CIM are fatigue, low-grade fever, poor appetite, head-ache, muscle aches, and swollen lymph nodes. Also, depression, speech impairment, poor learning, school failure, and decreased motivation have been reported.

There is, on the other side of the controversy, a larger body of specialists who say that all of these symptoms are found in many other physical and emotional disorders and that the existence of CIM has not yet been proven. A diagnosis of CIM is appealing because it gives an organic explanation for many complaints that are so often thought to be due to emotional stress or to be psychological in nature. The issue is still unresolved, and studies are continuing.

Requests from doctors that a child be excused from PE or receive home-bound teaching should be dealt with individually. If there is any question about complying with the physician's request, the school nurse and principal will require some assistance from a physician consultant or a specialist in infectious diseases.

VIRAL HEPATITIS

Nature of the Condition

Hapatitis means inflammation of the liver. It can be caused by chemicals, viruses, bacteria, fungi, or other agents. Whatever the cause, the symptoms are:

1. Early: fever, malaise (feeling sick), loss of appetite, and stom-achache.

2. One to two days later: continuation of early symptoms, plus nausea and vomiting.

3. About the same time or one to two days later: jaundice and enlarged liver.

Most children do not have all of the above symptoms. The severity is usually age related—children have a milder form of the disease. Therefore, many children develop *anicteric hepatitis* (*icterus* means jaundice); they have the disease but no jaundice. The whites of the eyes offer the easiest and earliest place to detect yellow discoloration. A child with very mild disease may have only a three to five day illness with low fever, loss of appetite, nausea, and a little stomachache; then the child gets well. Many of these children don't even stay home from school, and nobody ever knows they had hepatitis. They are, of course, just as contagious.

Varieties

There are two major types of viral hepatitis that are of school concern:

1. *Infectious hepatitis,* or hepatitis A, caused by the hepatitis A Virus (HAV)
2. *Serum hepatitis,* or hepatitis B, caused by the hepatitis B virus (HBV)

Hepatitis A

Almost all cases in school children are of this type. It is caused by oral ingestion of HAV. Transmission is by the fecal-oral route. Human sewage or fecal material which contains the virus and enters the water or food supply is a source of infection. Also, people with virus in their stools transmit it by way of their fingers (failure to wash hands after a bowel movement). A reservoir of viral hepatitis A exists in day-care centers catering to children under the age of two years (obviously related to diaper changing).

The incubation period (the time between ingestion of the virus and the earliest onset of symptoms) is fifteen to forty-five days.

The most contagious stage is in the late incubation period, so that by the time jaundice develops and the diagnosis is made, the disease is rapidly becoming less contagious, even though the patient may be getting sicker.

Half of the population over the age of fifty has antibodies against hepatitis A, meaning that they had the disease at some earlier time in their lives. One attack usually confers lifetime immunity, and there are no chronic carriers. Rarely is the disease severe, and the overall mortality rate is less than 1 percent. There are no healthy carriers.

Hepatitis B

Hepatitis B is caused by a completely different virus which can be found in blood, urine, feces, semen, vaginal secretions, saliva, breast milk, and other body fluids of infected individuals.

It was previously thought to occur only following blood transfusions and was called serum hepatitis. Now, because of blood donor screening, it is rarely transmitted this way. The most common methods of spread are by homo- and heterosexual contact and by intravenous drug abuse. Thus, there is a high prevalence among prostitutes, especially those who are IV drug abusers. Homosexual males also have high prevalence rates. There is a slightly higher prevalence in health care workers, especially some lab technicians, surgeons and dentists.

Hepatitis B, in contrast to A, has a much longer incubation period, one to six months, and chronic carriers are common; thus, it is thought that there is a pool of about one million active carriers in the United States. Since the symptoms of the active disease are similar to those of hepatitis A, sophisticated laboratory work and good clinical detection are required to be able to tell one from the other.

The following chart summarizes the major differences between A and B:

	HEPATITIS A	HEPATITIS B
Incubation Period	4–6 weeks	1–6 months
Period of Infectivity	short	may be long
Clinical Symptoms	same	same
Carrier State	no	yes

Laboratory Differentiation of Hepatitis A and B

There are two basic types of laboratory tests:

1. *Liver Function Tests*
   A. Bilirubin level
   B. SGOT (serum glutamic oxalate transaminase)
      SGPT (serum glutamic pyruvic transaminase)

Transaminase measures the degree of liver dysfunction (the more dysfunction, the higher the transaminase). Bilirubin measures the degree of jaundice (more jaundice, higher bilirubin). Both tests are equally abnormal in hepatitis A and B; they cannot be used to differentiate.

2. Antigen/Antibody Tests

    A. For hepatitis A. Hepatitis A antibodies (Anti-HA) can be detected following the onset of clinical disease (fever and jaundice). Their presence confirms type A infection. Other tests are available for earlier detection, but they are expensive and difficult to do.

    B. For hepatitis B. There are three separate hepatitis B antigens. Each produces its own antibody. Clinical labs refer to all six collectively as *"Hepatitis B antibody profile."*

1. Hepatitis B surface antigen	HBsAg*
Hepatitis B surface antibody	Anti-HBs
2. Hepatitis B core antigen	HBcAg
Hepatitis B core antibody	Anti-HBc
3. Hepatitis B e antigen	HBeAg
Hepatitis B e antibody	Anti-HBe

By a judicious selection of which of the six antigen/antibody tests, and by the clinical condition of the patient (sick vs. well, illness recently or long ago), the doctor can determine whether the patient has active infection, is a carrier, is infectious, and what precautions need be taken. Most physicians will consult with a specialist in infectious diseases.

Unless antigen/antibody studies are performed, it is impossible to be sure whether any one person with hepatitis has A or B. However, since a hepatitis antibody profile is expensive, and since the large majority of children with mild hepatitis have the A variety, doctors often only do the liver function tests and make a *clinical* diagnosis (as opposed to laboratory diagnosis) of hepatitis A. Most state Health Departments require a doctor's diagnosis, but do not dictate what criteria must be used in arriving at that diagnosis. Many doctors will

---

* When one tests an asymptomatic hepatitis B carrier, the usual result is: HBsAg-Positive.

order hepatitis B antibody profiles only if they suspect child sexual abuse or if the disease is unusually severe.

Treatment

There is no specific treatment for viral hepatitis. There is no antibiotic or antiviral medicine that actually kills the virus; therefore, preventive measures are of paramount importance.

There are many supportive measures that are helpful:

1. *Rest.* In the early stages it is important for children to be in bed or at least indoors, depending on the severity of the disease.

2. *Food.* Since loss of appetite and nausea are prominent symptoms, it is difficult for the child to eat the foods necessary to fortify the liver. Small amounts of appetizing carbohydrates at frequent intervals are helpful.

3. *Fluids.* All types of liquids are helpful, and in the early stages of the illness the child may not tolerate much else without vomiting.

Prevention of Hepatitis A

Handwashing

If everyone always washed hands after a bowel movement and if no one ever put their hands to their faces, childhood hepatitis would diminish markedly. Handwashing is by far the most effective way to prevent the spread of hepatitis A, especially after visits to the bathroom. Unfortunately, in spite of all exhortations, this practice is not followed, and there is no reason to expect that education alone can be relied on.

Gamma Globulin (GG), Now Called Immune Globulin (IG)

Hepatitis A can be prevented about 90 percent of the time if a dose of 0.02 cc of IG per kilogram of body weight is given intramuscularly within two weeks of exposure. This means that a 150 lb. individual would require a dose of about $1\frac{1}{2}$ cc. In some cases, larger doses are used because the doctor may suspect hepatitis B, which requires a dose three times larger, or because exposure occurred more than two weeks before the shot is given.

Prevention of Hepatitis B

Prevention of hepatitis B consists of taking the same measures recommended to prevent AIDS. In addition, there is now available an effective vaccine that permanently prevents hepatitis B, plus a special hepatitis B immune globulin. It is expensive, but it is recommended for high-risk individuals. A physician should make the decision as to who should receive it.

School Relevance

How Frequent and How Dangerous Is Hepatitis

Hepatitis is a low incidence disease. In a school of 500 students, for example, there will rarely be more than three to five cases a year. Many teachers and school administrators view hepatitis with more fear than it deserves. It is true that there are fatal cases, but these are rare; there are more fatalities from measles. Many teachers are immune to hepatitis because of minimal contact with the virus in childhood. Also, an understanding of how it is transmitted should allay the fears expressed by teachers and parents. Because of the method of transmission, it is unlikely that anyone will catch it at school. Most cases seen in school are caught at home four to six weeks earlier.

Cleaning of Classrooms

Some schools institute a massive cleaning program each time a case of hepatitis is discovered in the school. While it may help to wash doorknobs, handles, and other objects that are customarily touched, it doesn't help to scrub floors or spray walls or rooms. This is expensive, and some sprays are actually dangerous.

Reporting to Parents and Health Department

In most states, hepatitis is a reportable disease. Confirmed cases should be reported to the local public health authorities. Some school districts send notices to parents when a case occurs. This allows parents to seek advice from a doctor or the school nurse when they learn their child may have been exposed. (See the sample informative letter in Figure 8–1.)

Who Gets Immune Globulin

The question of whether to give school contacts a shot of IG always arises. The answer is usually no if the exposure is only in the classroom. For special close friends who play together every day, or for siblings, the doctor usually suggests that it be given. There are two things to remember.

First, each case is individual, and the child's personal physician should make the decision. There are many extenuating circumstances that go into the final decision of whether or not to administer IG and how much to give.

Second, most school-contact children do not need it. The American Academy of Pediatrics (AAP) does not recommend that IG be administered unless a school-centered epidemic occurs.

HEPATITIS

Dear Parent:

A case of hepatitis has occurred in your child's classroom. We have taken the precautionary measures prescribed by the public health authorities to prevent the spread of the disease. Hepatitis is a disease that is not very contagious (compared to measles, etc.), and therefore it is unusual for two cases to occur in the same classroom. It is usually mild in children. It is caused by a virus or germ that may be found in secretions of the mouth and nose, but is especially found in the urine and stool of the person with the disease. Therefore, washing the hands after going to the bathroom is especially important.

Protection with gamma globulin is recommended only for certain household contacts and people living in institutions such as orphanages or state hospitals.

If you have reason to believe that your child was exposed more intimately (spending the night at the home of the sick child, best friend, etc.), or if you have any other doubts or special questions, please call your family physician or contact the school nurse.

Figure 8–1.

The AAP has recommendations for the use of IG in day care centers. Since many children of day care age are now in public schools, these recommendations will be available for school nurses when they are counseling teachers and principals:

IG FOR DAY CARE CENTERS

In centers with all children more than two years old or who are toilet trained: when a case of hepatitis A is identified in an employee or enrolled child, IG is recommended for all employees and all children in the same room as the index case.

In day care centers with children not yet toilet trained: when one case of HAV infection is identified in a child or employee, or in the household contacts of two of the enrolled children, IG (0.02 ml/kg) is recommended for all employees and enrolled children. During the six weeks after the last case is identified, new employees and children also should receive IG. If recognition of the day care center outbreak is delayed by three or more weeks from the onset of the index case, or illness already has occurred in three or more families, wide spread of the disease is likely to have occurred already. In this situation, IG should be considered for use in all the day care staff and children and for the household contacts of all enrolled children who are 3 years old or younger.
(From *Red Book on Infectious Diseases* American Academy of Pediatrics, 1986., P.O. Box 927, Elk Grove Village, IL 60007.)

REYE SYNDROME

Reye Syndrome (RS) was first described by an Australian physician, Dr. R. D. K. Reye, in 1963. It occurs almost exclusively in children under age eighteen; the peak incidence is between six and ten years of age. It occurs equally in boys and girls and is more common in whites.

Symptoms

RS usually occurs following recovery from an acute viral illness, especially influenza or chicken pox. About one to three days after the fever from the viral illness, severe vomiting begins and lasts twelve to twenty-four hours. This is rapidly followed by lethargy, disorientation, combativeness, body stiffness, and coma of varying degrees. The progression to severe coma may stop at any point; the more rapid and severe the coma and stiffness, the worse the prognosis.

Differential Diagnosis

RS may be mistaken for acute viral encephalitis or hepatitis, diabetic acidosis, lead poisoning, or theophylline intoxication. These conditions can be rapidly diagnosed if they are kept in mind and tested for.

Pathology

The mitochondria (tiny structures inside the cell) are affected in all body organs, but there is no evidence of bacterial or virus infection. Body protein and fat are broken down at a rapid rate, the liver cells become filled with fat droplets and thus fail to function properly. The brain becomes water logged and swells up, causing increased intra-cranial pressure.

The symptoms are largely due to the liver failure, brain swelling, and rapid breakdown of body protein.

The characteristic blood test is a high level of ammonia.

Relationship to Aspirin

It is now universally accepted that aspirin plays some role in causing RS. Salicylates are capable of causing mitochondrial dysfunction, and this may be the trigger that causes RS in susceptible children.

All authorities recommend that children not be given aspirin to reduce the fever of any viral illness, especially influenza or chicken pox. If something must be given for discomfort associated with fever, acetaminophen (Tylenol™) is recommended.

School Relevance

In the past five to ten years, the peak age incidence of RS has been going up. Whereas the peak age used to be seven, it is now about ten in some published cases, and there is a suspicion that this is due to children medicating themselves with aspirin for minor illnesses. Many children with minor viral infections take aspirin without consulting their parents. This is an area in which school nurses can team with health education teachers and, with poster displays and other teaching aids, acquaint middle and high school students with the facts about RS.

REPORTED CASES OF REYE SYNDROME (RS) UNITED STATES, 1974 AND 1977–1988

Year	RS Cases
1974	379
1977	454
1978	236
1979	389
1980	555
1981	297
1982	213
1983	198
1984	204
1985	93
1986	101

MMWR, October 23, 1987, Vol. 36/No. 41

VENEREAL DISEASE

Modern society talks about and engages in sexual practices more than in the past. Promiscuity has affected the student population as well. More individuals are sexually active at a younger age and with a greater variety of partners. This has caused venereal disease (VD) to leap to epidemic numbers. Whereas in the past VD meant syphilis and gonorrhea, the rapidly rising number of cases has caused previously rare conditions to be added to the list of sexually transmitted diseases.

Herpes simplex, hepatitis B, and several lesser-known diseases are seen more and more often.

In spite of the serious threat this presents to schoolchildren, there is still widespread opposition to presenting effective education in the schools to offer the students information that could protect them from such exposure. The assumption is that if the students hear about sex, they will get ideas. In actual fact, they have already heard about it. Lots of them are past the idea stage. Those students who are not sexually active have made the choice for abstinence in spite of the fact that they have heard about sex. How simple it would be if society could view VD as dispassionately as it now does tuberculosis! Then methods of reporting and treating existing cases would become more effective, causing the incidence to drop.

Sex Education

Unfortunately, too many current attempts at sex education resemble the scare tactics used in the late 1960s and early 1970s which tried to dissuade young people from using marijuana. A common approach to sex education is to invite a guest speaker from some agency to show a film during gym to some forty to sixty students of the same sex. The movie preaches sexual abstinence, depicts the horrors of various venereal diseases, and describes the treatment for these illnesses. This is followed by a question-and-answer period. Unfortunately, this message has not had the desired effect in junior and senior high schools, where the prevalence of venereal disease remains high. It is doubtful that current health education methods will work. To be effective, this type of education will have to embrace the wider area of sexuality in general, consider the negative aspects of recreational sex and emphasize emotional love and responsibility over hormonal urges. Above all, it will have to be built on some simple, basic knowledge of anatomy and physiology. This will not happen until society urges schools to incorporate this kind of teaching, beginning in the elementary grades, and until colleges begin training teachers who can teach it. In addition, unless TV and radio reinforce this message, the school teaching will be only minimally effective.

Such effective sex education will help control not only venereal disease, but many other problems connected with contemporary sexual practices.

School Relevance

Obviously, it is never necessary to exclude a pupil from school because of VD, even in the unlikely event that its existence should become known. None of the other students or faculty is in danger of contracting the disease in a nonvenereal way.

Relating to Health Department

Frequently, the local health department, in its case-finding efforts, will contact a school official to report that one of the students in that school has been named as a contact. This often happens when another student, following the appearance of certain alarming symptoms, goes directly to the health department for diagnosis and treatment, not only bypassing the family physician, but the family as well. The law now permits the health department to treat these youngsters without parental consent. In the course of treatment the infected youngster is asked to name all of the sexual contacts involved so that they can be warned or treated, as the case may be. The health department, to keep the youngster's confidence and preserve his or her privacy, often tries to talk to the named contact at school rather than at home. (Also, it's easier to find children at school.)

Often the principal is troubled by someone from outside the school talking to a student about such matters without the parents being aware of what's happening. Naturally, it's better for all concerned if the student is able to tell the parents what has happened and to have them cooperate in the treatment. However, as every principal knows, there are many homes in which this type of communication simply cannot and does not take place. In such circumstances, it is far better to have the youngster adequately treated because of the potential dangers of ravaging complications. The principal should arrange a private room where the venereal disease control agent from the health department can talk to the student personally, or arrange a quiet, private, and confidential telephone conversation and then use his or her influence or that of the counselor or school nurse to urge the student to obtain the necessary tests for diagnosis and treatment.

Routes of Transmission

In spite of the fact that it is theoretically possible for any venereal disease to be transmitted by nonvenereal means, in actual practice is is rare for an individual to contact any venereal disease other than by some form of direct sexual activity—in particular, direct mouth-to-mouth kissing or direct genital contact, either heterosexual or homosexual. Contracting venereal disease from a toilet seat or drinking glass or any other intermediate object is largely a myth; it is theoretically possible and undoubtedly some cases exist, but few have been documented outside of the laboratory worker who accidentally pricks his or her finger with a needle containing infected blood or serum.

SYPHILIS

Nature of the Condition

Syphilis has plagued humankind since antiquity. It has existed for so many centuries that it seems the human race has developed a partial immunity to it. Several hundred years ago, *spirocheta pallida*, the germ that causes syphilis, was so virulent that it occasionally caused a high fever, delirium, coma, and death within a week. In recent years, the prevalence rates have been increasing, and more cases will be seen in schoolchildren.

Symptoms and Stages

Primary

The primary lesion usually consists of a genital sore (chancre) that goes away untreated in one to three weeks. There may or may not be a low-grade fever, but the affected individual is not very sick. Since the chancre is relatively painless, the doctor is often not even consulted, although the disease is highly contagious. The chancre is usually located on the glans penis (the tip end), the labia minora (the inner vaginal lips), and rarely on the tonsil or adjacent to the rectal opening.

Secondary

The secondary stage of syphilis occurs about six to eight weeks later and can manifest itself in various forms. A common finding is a nonitching skin rash that looks like mild measles. Whitish patches sometimes occur inside the mouth and are called *mucus patches*. They are highly contagious, especially through kissing. This stage is usually accompanied by fever and malaise. It usually goes away untreated in one to three weeks. There are many other possible manifestations of secondary syphilis, such as acute meningitis or encephalitis, different kinds of skin rashes, bald spots, and arthritis. Occasionally, secondary symptoms continue to reappear for six to nine months or for as long as two years.

Tertiary

The first two stages are almost always benign and self-limiting. The third or tertiary stage occurs five to twenty years later. It has become quite rare since the availability of penicillin. The tertiary stage in untreated syphilis occurs in only about 25 to 30 percent of individuals who have had the primary or secondary stage. It can attack the brain, spinal cord, heart, or other organs. In any case, the illness and damage caused by the tertiary stage are usually serious and sometimes fatal.

TREATMENT

The treatment today is extremely simple and effective. The first effective treatment was a form of arsenic developed by Paul Ehrlich. It was called salvarsan, was quite toxic, required a two- to three-year course of treatment, and did not work too well. Treatment methods were gradually refined and arsenic preparations improved, so that by about 1940 one could cure many cases of early syphilis (primary or secondary) with a six-month course of quite painful injections of a new type of arsenic and bismuth. Nowadays, most early syphilis can be cured dependably with a single shot of the proper dose of penicillin. This represents one of the most dramatic miracle cures ever wrought by medical science.

GONORRHEA

Nature of the Condition

Gonorrhea, now one of the most common communicable disease in the world except for the common cold, is also one of the classical venereal diseases of antiquity. It is commonly called *the clap* and is caused by a germ called *Neisseria gonorrhea* or simply the gonococcus. It settles in the urethra in males and in the cervix in females, producing a purulent (pus) discharge plus various other symptoms. The time between exposure and first onset of symptoms can be two to ten days, but in most cases it is about two to four days.

Symptoms

In males this infection causes burning on urination. In females the infection is often painless, but if it spreads up into the uterus and fallopian tubes, it can cause intense abdominal pain. Further serious complications such as peritonitis may ensue if treatment is delayed. Also, complications can occur in males, especially if the infection travels to the testicles or prostate gland.

In recent years the gonococcus has been found in the throat and rectum in increasing numbers of patients who regularly indulge in oral or anal sex practices, either homosexual or heterosexual.

In both males and females, either because of partial natural immunity or partial treatment, the urethral or vaginal discharge can diminish to such a small amount that it is almost unnoticeable and completely painless. It is, however, just as contagious. Gonorrhea has become unchallenged as the most prevalent of all serious venereal diseases, and the incidence is rising each year.

Treatment

Treatment is quite simple; a single injection of penicillin will cure most early cases, but most physicians prescribe a combination of medications. The gonococcus tends to develop a resistance against antibiotic action, and many strains of the germ are partially or completely penicillin-resistant. If complications ensue, a longer course of treatment is usually required, along with bed rest.

NONSPECIFIC URETHRITIS AND OTHER GENITAL INFECTIONS

Nature of the Condition

In addition to the gonococcus, there are many germs, viruses, and fungi that can cause infections in the urethra, vagina, cervix, or other genital organs. Taken as a group, infections with any of these agents have been labeled nonspecific urethritis or nonspecific genital disease. In some cases, the causative organism can be identified.

At the present time, the known causative agents of genito-urinary disease, all of which are capable of being spread by sexual contact are:

1. *Trichomonas*—a one-celled animal organism (related to the amoeba)
2. *Monilia*—a yeast-like fungus
3. *Chlamydia*—a combination virus-bacterium
4. *Herpes simplex*—a pure virus

The first three of the above cause only a mild vaginal or urethral discharge. The fourth—herpes virus—causes sores that burn or itch. This is the same virus that causes fever blisters around the nose and lips and can also cause similar sores on the penis (usually the tip end) or around the cervix. These sores itch and burn and are readily spread by sexual contact. In addition to the burning and itching, it is suspected that women with herpes infections of the cervix are more prone to develop cancer of the cervix.

Symptoms

Generally speaking, these diseases usually cause a mild urethral or vaginal discharge, some itching, plus a small amount of burning on urination. In almost all cases, the degree of symptoms is less than in gonorrhea. Also, complications rarely occur. Since a small amount of vaginal discharge is normal, a woman with a very mild nonspecific vaginitis may be unaware of her infection yet fully capable of passing it on to her sexual partner. Also, the male can unknowingly harbor certain organisms in his urethra without developing any noticeable symptoms but be capable of infecting his sexual partner. A married couple may continue to give the infection to each other unless both are treated simultaneously, even though only one (usually the female) may manifest symptoms.

There are two types of herpes virus. Type I is found about the nose and lips, type II in the genital area. They can be differentiated with certain laboratory tests, and it is now known that type I virus can also infect the genital area with oral-genital contact. (See Section 2)

With good methods of detection, the cause can be identified in about 60 to 70 percent of all cases of mild genitourinary infection. That leaves 30 to 40 percent of nonspecific disease for which no cause can be found.

Treatment

Treatment varies depending on the causative organism. Chlamydia, trichomonas, and monilia can all be treated quite effectively. There is as yet no effective cure for herpes infection, although many agents have been tried. The remaining venereal diseases, those that are truly nonspecific (cause unknown), are treated by cleanliness, time, and educated guesses.

OTHER VENEREAL DISEASES

Nature of the Condition

Diseases spread by venereal contact, in the United States as in other parts of the world, exist in larger numbers than many people are aware. Some experts claim there are about twenty. The less common are unknown to most people, and the average doctor rarely sees them. They are commonly seen in VD clinics.

Generally speaking, they cause various kinds of surface lesions (sores, warts, lymph node swellings, etc.) in the genital area, and occasionally more serious complications ensue. Some of these diseases are:

- Lymphogranuloma venereum
- Chancroid (soft chancre)
- Venereal warts
- Granuloma inguinale
- Reiter's disease
- Hepatitis B
- AIDS (acquired immune deficiency syndrome)

Some of the less common venereal diseases are readily treatable, and some are not. In all cases, a specialist in venereal diseases needs to be consulted.

CHRONIC TRANSMISSIBLE NEONATAL INFECTIONS

CHRONIC TRANSMISSIBLE NEONATAL INFECTIONS

Nature of the Condition

The fetus and newborn are susceptible to many infections during pregnancy, during the birth process, or shortly after birth. A small number of these diseases are capable of causing a long-term illness that may be contagious even as the child grows older and enters school.

Most of these infections are due to viruses, including the following:

- Cytomegalovirus (CMV)
- Rubella virus (RV)
- Varicella-zoster virus (VZV)
- Herpes simplex virus (HSV)
- Hepatitis B virus (HBV)

The chart in Figure 9–1 from *Textbook of Pediatric Infectious Diseases* (edited by R. D. Feigin and J. D. Cherry, Chapter 21 by James C. Overall, Jr.; Philadelphia: W. B. Saunders, 1981) provides a graphic description of different ways the virus can spread from the mother to the newborn, and how it may cause a persistent infection in the infant.

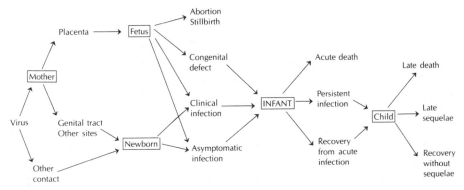

Figure 9–1

Viral infection calls forth an antibody response, and measuring the antibody level is the usual laboratory method of determining whether a person has had the disease in the past.

When adults are infected by these viruses, it is rarely serious. However, if a woman gets one of these diseases while she is pregnant, she may transmit the virus to her fetus. *This is precisely why school personnel have become so concerned.*

School Relevance

Many physically and mentally disabled students, some profoundly so, are now in public schools. It is known that some of the diseases described above can cause infection of the brain and other organs in the fetus and newborn, which later may result in physical and mental retardation. The primary concern of school personnel is *how long these babies may remain contagious.* These are legitimate concerns for which there are, most of the time, dependable answers.

For example, a baby whose brain has been damaged by HSV is obviously contagious as long as there are herpetic skin lesions. On the other hand, a newborn baby with a liver infection due to HBV may become a chronic hepatitis B carrier and be no more contagious than any other HB carrier (of whom there are always several in the school population of students and teachers).

CYTOMEGALOVIRUS

Cytomegalovirus (CMV) exists worldwide, and antibodies indicating past infection are found in 60 to 90 percent of the various populations tested. It is most commonly contracted during infancy and early childhood from the mother, and or during young adult life from sexual activity. There are several viral strains; immunity to one does not necessarily confer immunity to others. The virus can be recovered from urine, semen, saliva, and vaginal and other body secretions.

Acquisition of the virus rarely results in clinical disease, except in persons with a weak immune system. The groups at high risk of developing symptomatic illness are fetus and newborn, persons on immune suppressing drugs such as steroids (athletes take note!), and

AIDS patients. The remainder develop only an increased blood antibody level. A person who acquires the infection, though asymptomatic, may remain contagious for a long time. In addition, a person who has had the disease, developed antibodies, but whose body fluids no longer contain the virus, can get reinfected with another strain of CMV and become contagious again. It is easy to see why the distribution of the virus is so widespread.

Special Precautions in Pregnancy

Since CMV can be so devastating in the newborn, women who are pregnant or may soon become pregnant should take precautions to prevent exposure. In actual practice, this means no promiscuous, unprotected sexual activity, since this is the usual route of transmission in adults.

Young women working in day care centers can catch CMV from the children. Now that younger and more handicapped children are entering school, there is a greater risk of exposure, because caring for these children requires handling them. There is, as yet, no vaccine to prevent CMV or a medicine to cure it; the best prevention is hand washing. In-service educational programs by doctors or school nurses are useful. When school personnel have a clearer understanding of the disease, they cooperate better in hand washing and other preventive techniques.

Ninety to ninety-five percent of newborns with CMV are normal at birth. Those few showing signs of disease have a large spleen and liver and overt signs of brain damage. However, of the larger number of babies who have appeared to be normal at birth but whose blood test is CMV positive, long-term follow-up studies have shown this comparison (from *Textbook of Pediatric Infectious Diseases* by Feigin and Cherry):

Infected but normal infant		Noninfected normal infant
IQ under 90	32%	16%
hearing loss	23%	9%
predicted school		
failure	36%	14%
microcephaly	15%	5%

RUBELLA (GERMAN MEASLES)

German measles is, with rare exceptions, a barely noticeable, benign, three-day disease with a mild rash. However, contracting the disease during pregnancy, especially early pregnancy, often causes severe congenital malformations in the newborn. Also, 75 percent of the newborns who appear normal at birth but are born to mothers who had rubella during pregnancy, develop long-term sequelae (mild mental retardation, learning disability, clumsiness, etc.) in the first five years of life. Therefore, all women should be vaccinated against rubella in early life. Indeed, now that immunization is required for school entry in all states, there has not been a major rubella epidemic in the U.S. since 1964, and congenital malformations from rubella are rarely seen.

Recent surveys show that 5 to 20 percent of young women are susceptible to rubella. When a nonimmunized woman becomes pregnant, what should be done when (or if) she is exposed to rubella? The vaccine package insert states that it should not be given to pregnant women, or women about to become pregnant. However, about 1,200 such women in the U.S. have received the vaccine and no rubella babies have resulted. When this situation arises, each woman should be individually counseled by a physician.

A baby born with congenital malformations from maternal rubella is contagious, i.e., virus is being shed. Rubella babies may shed virus for as long as a year, but rarely, if ever, longer. Therefore, most school-age children will not be contagious, only some of those enrolling in 0–3 special programs.

Needless to say, all school personnel, especially women in their childbearing years, should be immunized. (In 1986, three cases of neonatal congenital rubella were reported in Texas, the first documented cases since 1981.)

VARICELLA AND ZOSTER (CHICKEN POX AND SHINGLES)

Varicella is chicken pox; *zoster* (also called herpes zoster) is shingles. The virus that causes both diseases is identical. When the body is first invaded by the varicella-zoster virus, (VZV), usually during childhood, chicken pox results. After recovery, the virus may remain in the body in a latent, noncontagious form. On re-exposure years later, the latent virus may become reactivated and, because of partial immunity, shingles develops. Shingles is a localized form of chicken pox.

Varicella is one of the most contagious of all diseases; 96 percent of susceptible contacts develop the disease within one month of exposure. Shingles is contagious only on close contact; exact figures are unavailable because the disease is uncommon.

Infection of a pregnant woman with VZV results in one of three syndromes in her baby:

1. Congenital malformations. These babies have no skin lesions and are not contagious, though they may have serious malformations of peripheral nerves, spinal cord, brain, and eyes.

2. Neonatal chicken pox. These babies may be gravely ill; the mortality rate is high. After they recover and the rash has gone, they are not contagious.

3. Shingles in infancy or childhood. These infections are usually not severe; they are mildly contagious only as long as the rash is active.

Obviously, school personnel need not be concerned. If a woman of childbearing age is concerned about her susceptibility to chicken pox, blood tests are available to check her antibody level. This is not recommended as a routine measure, since most adults are immune. A child with chicken pox will not be allowed to stay in school. A child with shingles will only be in school if the rash is slight and on a part of the body covered by clothing. If the shingles rash is exposed or if the child is sick, that is also reason for having the student stay at home. However, shingles can last several weeks or months, and in most cases, the child is not clinically ill with fever or other symptoms. It is safe to allow a child to attend school with shingles provided care is taken to keep the rash covered by clothing, especially during P.E.

HERPES SIMPLEX VIRUS

Cold sores or fever blisters are due to the herpes simplex virus (HSV). HSV and varicella-zoster virus (VZV) both belong to the herpes family of viruses, but they are separate and distinct; they only share the same first name. There are two types of HSV.

- Type I causes mouth, nose, and eye lesions (cold sores and fever blisters).
- Type II is a genital infection. (About 10 to 20 percent of the time genital herpes is caused by Type I virus and herpes sores on the face are caused by Type II.)

HSV can be transmitted by a pregnant woman to her baby in one of three ways:

1. In utero through the placenta.

2. During the birth process from active sores in the genital tract. Babies who get HSV in utero or during the birth process may develop a very severe form of the disease called *disseminated herpes*. The mortality rate is high, and those who live often have severe brain damage and may require diapering, feeding, or other manipulation.

3. After birth from a mother with active sores, either by direct contact or hand to mouth transmission.

School Relevance

How Contagious Are Children with Herpes?

Those with skin lesions are definitely contagious; those without skin lesions probably are not. Children who live long enough to enter school will be no more contagious than any child who has had herpes (cold sores) in early life. The HSV remains latent in the nerve roots of the spinal cord, and the child is contagious on direct contact whenever there is an outbreak of cold sores.

The children with neonatal herpes who survive often are mentally retarded and drool. Their saliva may be contagious when the child has active skin lesions, but not when the virus lies dormant in the spinal cord.

INFANT HEPATITIS B

HBV can be transmitted to the *fetus* through the placenta; to the *newborn* during the birth process; or *postnatally* by exposure to the mother or others.

Most babies born with HBV, or who get it postnatally, have mothers who are asymptomatic hepatitis B carriers. The babies are also often asymptomatic carriers, having neither fever nor jaundice. Some remain carriers for a short period of time, and some for a long period—months or years. A small percentage (6 to 10 percent) may get a severe or fatal disease.

It is estimated that about 10 percent of the general population are chronic hepatitis B carriers. The various types of carriers, their contagiousness, and school relevance are discussed fully in Chapter 8.

TOXOPLASMOSIS

Toxoplasmosis is a widespread disease, caused by a one-celled organism (germ), toxoplasma gondi. Cats are the natural host of this disease, but humans (and animals other than cats) become infected by exposure to cat feces (changing the litter box) or by eating meat of other infected animals.

Although prevalent, it rarely causes noticeable symptoms of illness when first acquired. Once antibodies develop, it can be detected by a blood test. If a woman first acquires the infection while pregnant, she can pass the active disease on to her fetus, which may result in fetal brain or eye damage. In a school for the blind, a small population may well be children with congenital toxoplasmosis. Most of these children are also mentally retarded.

School Relevance

Infants and children who had the disease are *not* contagious; there is no danger that a pregnant teacher could get the disease from a student. The disease is discussed here because some young children with congenital toxoplasmosis are often placed in early childhood special education classes. The nurse can reassure others that this student is no threat, and she can suggest further investigation for those children who have not been diagnosed.

SECTION 10

BITES AND STINGS

Bees and Wasps
- Nature of the Condition
- Symptoms
  —Local Reactions
  —Generalized Reactions

Fire Ants and Other Insects

Spiders

Human Bites

BEES AND WASPS

Nature of the Condition

The most common insect stings are those of bees, wasps, yellow jackets, and fire ants—all members of the *hymenoptera* family. These stings usually cause a severe pain that diminishes over five to ten minutes, and in fifteen minutes the symptoms have all but gone. While the amount of pain and swelling varies with each individual sting, the types of reactions fall into two major categories.

Symptoms

Local Reactions

This type of reaction indicates that the body's immune mechanism is effectively defending against the insect venom and thereby preventing the entire body from reacting adversely. Following are some examples:

1. A small, red, painful, swollen area that becomes normal in ten to fifteen minutes
2. A sting on the hand or foot, causing equal duration of pain, but with the entire hand or foot remaining swollen for several days
3. A sting on the forehead that causes both eyes to swell

Generalized Reactions

These occur in a part of the body far removed from the bite. Examples are swelling of the lips and/or eyelids from a bite on the hand, a rash all over the body from a single sting anywhere, or swelling of the hands from a bite on the leg. Reactions of this nature can be dangerous because they indicate that the body has a weak immune mechanism against insect venom and signal the possibility of an increasingly severe reaction to subsequent stings. In the United States, there are about fifty to sixty deaths a year from bee or wasp stings; they are almost all caused by one of the following severe types of generalized reactions:

1. *Swelling of the larynx* (voice box), the narrowest part of the airway. A small degree of swelling can cause obstruction to respiration.

2. *Anaphylactic shock* resulting when all of the small blood vessels in the body dilate and cause the blood pressure to drop very quickly. The patient suddenly feels faint, begins to perspire, feels cold, and in a very short time may lose consciousness.

Treatment and School Relevance

The school principal and school nurse should see that the playground and buildings are periodically inspected, and the students should be instructed to report any beehives, wasp nests or fire ant mounds. Local reactions are best treated with an ice cube or an anesthetic ointment like benzocaine. Another useful household remedy is meat tenderizer that contains an enzyme derived from papaya. (This is also useful to relieve jellyfish or Portuguese man-o'-war stings.) Juice of the aloe vera plant has also been recommended.

If the stinger is present, it should be removed with the fingernail or a knife blade. Since it usually has a tiny venom sac attached, care must be taken not to squeeze it.

In cases of persistent swelling of the hands or feet because of local reactions, it is best to consult a doctor. Though medicine taken internally is rarely necessary for local reactions, on occasion it may be required.

Since generalized reactions are always potentially serious, it is advisable to consult a physician. Most allergists recommend a series of desensitization shots and in addition request that the patient carry a small kit containing adrenalin, an antihistamine, and a needle and syringe. (See Figure 10–1.) With proper prevention and treatment, almost all severe or fatal reactions can be avoided.

The school principal should allow this kit to be kept in a refrigerator and should make it readily accessible to the child, the school nurse, or whoever is designated to give the injection when necessary. In cases of this nature it is well to establish contact with the child's physician. A sample form follows in Figure 10–2.

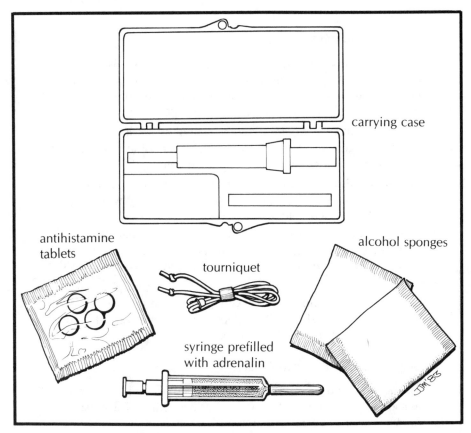

carrying case

antihistamine tablets

tourniquet

alcohol sponges

syringe prefilled with adrenalin

Figure 10–1. Emergency insect sting kit

GUIDELINES FOR EMERGENCY SCHOOL TREATMENT

**Emergency Medication—Injectable and/or Oral
For Extreme and Dangerous Hypersensitivity to Insect Sting**

Extreme hypersensitivity to insect sting is a potentially life-threatening situation. Many physicians ask these patients to carry an emergency kit containing injectable adrenalin (epinephrin) and/or an oral medicine.

Since this problem is rare but potentially extremely dangerous, we urge school district superintendents, school nurses, and physicians to be aware of the problem and, to as full an extent as possible, follow the proposed suggestions.

(continued)

I. Suggestions to the School District

1. The school district should accept an emergency insect sting kit prescribed by a physician if certain conditions are met as outlined below. The emergency kit should be kept where the child and a responsible adult can reach it fast.

2. The school district should allow the school nurse, if the nurse is on campus, to give an emergency injection at school in cases when the physican has met certain criteria outlined below.

3. The school district should allow the child to give himself or herself the injection if it has been properly prescribed and the physican has met the criteria outlined below.

4. Other campus personnel, previously identified as capable of giving shots, may be allowed to give the emergency injection if the school nurse is absent and the child cannot give it to himself or herself.

5. If the school nurse is not present, the child cannot give himself or herself the medication, and nobody is available to give it, the child should be evacuated by EMS or other more feasible method as soon as he or she reports having been stung.

II. Suggestions for the School Nurse

1. The nurse should give the injectable and/or oral medicine, as ordered, as soon as the child reports he or she has been stung. The nurse should not wait to observe any reactions.

2. The school nurse should recommend that the child be evacuated as soon as possible after the first dose of oral and/or injectable medicine.

3. If the child has not yet been evacuated, in 15 minutes the school nurse may give a second dose of oral and/or injectable medication provided it has been so prescribed by the physician.

III. Suggestions for the Physician

1. The school nurse will follow your orders as closely as the state Nurse Practice Act permits.

2. The school nurse can give emergency medication—oral and/or injectable—if school district policy permits.

3. The school nurse *cannot* observe a child for symptoms and then make a decision about whether to give or withhold oral or injectable medication. The nurse must give the medication immediately upon report of the sting and at such times (10 to 15 minutes) immediately after as prescribed.

(continued)

4. It is strongly recommended that the physician notify the school principal by telephone in each case, explain the situation, and ask to have the school nurse call back.

5. The physician must sent short, clear written instructions with each emergency kit in addition to the above phone call.

SAMPLE RECOMMENDATIONS FROM DOCTOR'S OFFICE TO ACCOMPANY INSECT ALLERGY EMERGENCY KIT

_____(name)_____ is highly allergic to the stings of bees, wasps, and ants and needs the following emergency care when stung:

1. Chew two tablets of chlortrimeton.

2. Give shot:_____cc of adrenalin.

3. Remove stinger if obvious. Remove the stinger from the wound if it is still present. Use fine tweezers, long fingernails, or a knife blade to scrape off the stinger. Do not grasp any fleshy portion of the venom sack, for it will inject more venom.

4. Use ice pads. Apply an ice pack, if available, to slow the absorption.

5. Go to emergency room or doctor's office.

6. Give second shot—same dose—in 15 minutes if still at school.

Please review these instructions every two or three months and check the epinephrin (adrenalin) at that time. Check expiration date. It must be replaced if any color develops or particles appear in the fluid. Refrigeration is not necessary, but avoid prolonged exposure to heat, such as in a closed car or in direct sun.

Do not discard the syringe or medicine vials, but take them with you to the emergency room or doctor's office in order that they can be sure of exactly what you've done.

Please call our office and report results of stings.

Figure 10–2.

FIRE ANTS AND OTHER INSECTS

This mound-building ant is found mostly in the southern warmer states. While the bite is quite painful, it rarely causes the serious generalized type of reaction described above. A small child could inadvertently stand in the ant bed and receive so many bites that the total envenomation would be serious. Fatalities are rare in people and animals.

Many caterpillars cause a sting via venom on their feet. The sting is painful and leaves a row of tiny blisters with a red base. These insects are called *urticating* (blister forming) caterpillars. Earwigs, scorpions, and other miscellaneous insects also bite and sting.

Treatment is always the same as for local reactions to bee stings. In cases of multiple fire ant bites, especially in a small child, immediate consultation with a physician is advisable.

SPIDERS

Spiders (not technically insects) rarely bite humans. Two that are of concern are the brown recluse and the black widow. Both types of bites should be referred to a physician as promptly as possible. Ice should be applied at school.

HUMAN BITES

Because of the large number of bacteria that live in the mouth, human bites—more than any other—are likely to become infected. Therefore, gentle washing, preferably with an antibacterial soap such as Septisol, is necessary. Following thorough cleansing, a loose dressing should be applied so that air can reach the abraded surface.

If the bite is minimal, daily washing will suffice to cure it. If it is worse, it should be referred to a physician.

SECTION 11

DIABETES

Diabetes
- Nature of the Condition
- Symptoms
  - —Type I: Juvenile Onset
  - —Type II: Adult Onset
- Diagnosis
- Special Problems at Adolescence and Emotional Problems
- Insulin, Diet, and Exercise
- Complications
- School Relevance and Role of the School Nurse
  - —Diet and Exercise
  - —Monitoring of Blood and Urine Sugar
  - —Family and Physician Contact

DIABETES

Nature of the Condition

Diabetes mellitus, or sugar diabetes, is a disease of one part of the pancreas (sweetbreads in cattle), a gland located near the stomach. This part of the pancreas secretes two hormones: insulin and glucagon. These two hormones regulate the blood's sugar level; insulin causes the blood sugar level to go down, and glucagon causes it to go up.

Patients with diabetes do not produce enough insulin; therefore, their blood sugar level goes up. As the blood sugar level rises, other changes occur that, in childhood, cause rapidly progressive severe symptoms.

There are two types of diabetes: Type I or juvenile-onset diabetes, and Type II or adult-onset diabetes. On occasion an older person (over 35) will develop type I diabetes, and very rarely a child will develop type II diabetes. Type I may be seen at any age in childhood. The peak age of onset is eleven to thirteen years. The younger the child, the faster the disease progresses. It is rare in children under three years old.

Symptoms

Type I: Juvenile Onset

The classical symptoms are excessive thirst, urination, appetite, and weight loss. The symptoms can progress quite rapidly, so that in two to four weeks the child becomes thin and dehydrated, progressively weaker, and less responsive, with deep, rapid respirations and, if untreated, coma and death. Associated symptoms are blurred vision, bed wetting, itching, and skin infections.

In addition to the abnormal sugar metabolism, other changes occur in the large and small arteries and the peripheral nerves. These changes, however, take many years to develop and are rarely seen in school children.

Children who are destined to develop diabetes are rarely over-weight; diet or excessive sugar intake is not the cause. It is inherited as a genetic predisposition.

Type II: Adult Onset

This almost always occurs in middle or later life, is associated with diet and obesity, and progresses slowly. It is extremely rare in school-age children, so it will not be dealt with in this section.

Diagnosis

Diabetes is a rare disease, occurring in about one in 2,500 children under age fifteen. A classical case of childhood diabetes can usually be diagnosed by symptoms alone. The school nurse should be on the lookout for any child who loses weight, especially if he or she continues to eat well. Diabetic children always lose weight; they never simply fail to gain. Many preadolescent children gain weight very slowly—two to four pounds a year—so diabetes need not be suspected if a child simply fails to gain. Blood and urine sugar tests are always performed to confirm the diagnosis and to determine the severity of the disease. Many school nurses now have urine test paper strips, which can be used in suspicious cases.

Special Problems at Adolescence and Emotional Problems

As with any handicapped child, the rebellious adolescent diabetic also presents special problems. It is important for the school nurse to help the child during special situations in school. Teachers may need explanations for rest-room excuses for urine testing. Coaches need to know about the importance of regularity of exercise with little change from day to day (the more exercise, the less insulin required—within limits). The principal needs to make allowances for absences; by communication with the physician, the school nurse can help determine which absences are necessary.

Diabetic children who develop hypoglycemia (excessively low blood sugar) are likely to exhibit agressiveness, irritability, or other behavioral problems as their first symptoms. **Any unusual behavior in a child with diabetes should arouse suspicions that the child may have an imbalance of blood sugar.**

Insulin, Diet, and Exercise

Juvenile diabetics (Type I) always need insulin; the condition cannot be controlled by diet alone. Oral antidiabetic medications, so commonly used in Type II diabetes, should not be used.

The treatment triad consists of:

1. Insulin
2. Diet
3. Exercise

The amount of insulin required varies for each child but always depends on the caloric intake and the amount of exercise. The more food eaten, the more insulin required; the more exercise, the less insulin required.

Insulin. Most children with diabetes will receive two doses a day, both at home; one in the morning and the second between 4:00 and 5:00 P.M. The individual total daily dose will vary from 5 units to 75 or 90 units, depending on many factors. The doctor will determine each child's dose. The school nurse should be alert to events that may require a change in or elimination of a dose. *Warning:* It is always safer to give too little insulin than too much. Too little insulin results in a *slow* rise in blood sugar with relatively slow onset of serious symptoms. Too much insulin results in a rapid decline in blood sugar with relatively *rapid* onset of serious symptoms. Whether or not the school nurse is scheduled to give a child a prescribed dose of insulin each day (a rare situation), the nurse must always be able to contact the doctor or doctor's assistant if a situation arises that requires a change in the daily dose.

Diet. The childhood diabetic needs a carefully prescribed diet. It is important that the child not become obese; blood sugar levels are unstable in overweight diabetics. The caloric content should remain steady and only vary within prescribed limits, and the diet should be one that the child enjoys and eats willingly. Special health foods and so-called diabetic foods are never necessary. Missing a meal is not a reason for omitting an insulin dose. It is a reason for finding out why the meal was missed and consultation with the doctor's office. It is not good practice for the child to regularly eat too much and take more insulin to control the resultant rise in blood sugar. It makes the diabetes more difficult to control. At the same time, it is not emotionally healthy to forbid the after-football-game chocolate ice cream sundae that "all the other kids are having." This type of exception can be, and usually is, easily worked out in advance.

Exercise. In 1935, Dr. E. P. Joslin wrote:

> Exercise tends to lower the blood sugar in the diabetic. . . . the effect is so striking and so beneficial that exercise . . . is now accorded a prominent place in treatment. . . . Through muscular activity food tolerance improves and higher diets with smaller doses of insulin are possible. This is most strikingly shown in the much lower insulin requirement of diabetic children in summer camp as compared to the larger need when they are in school and relatively inactive.

These words are still true. While regular exercise is important, the preteen child's normal play activities are usually sufficient. It is not necessary to enroll in special exercise, karate, or soccer classes for the sake of the diabetes alone. On the other hand, a sedentary child needs to be encouraged to run, climb, and jump in normal play. Teenage children more often need organized physical activities. In all cases, common sense—with due regard for the child's physical and emotional health—should prevail. It is impossible to control diabetes with exercise alone; proper diet and insulin are necessary.

Complications

Hypoglycemia (low blood sugar) is by far the most frequent complication. It is caused by excess insulin in relation to diet and exercise. It comes on rapidly and needs to be managed early before the child loses consciousness.

The early warning signs are sweating, pallor, trembling, rapid pulse, and blurred vision. Later signs are confusion, disorientation, aggressiveness, and partial or complete unconsciousness. As in adults who are mistaken to be drunk, students may appear drugged. This is also called *insulin reaction.*

Preferred early treatment is a glass of milk or orange juice. Each contains just enough rapidly absorbable sugar to cause a proper and safe rise in blood sugar. If there is no observable response in five minutes, the child should chew a package of mints, which contains more sugar. If symptoms are not relieved in five to ten minutes, the student must be rushed to the nearest emergency medical facility.

An ideal situation is to have a blood sugar testing kit on each campus (See below.) A blood sugar reading of less than 60 will show that the student is having an insulin reaction instead of early diabetic acidosis.

Glucagon is commercially available and is excellent for the treatment of insulin reactions. It is given intramuscularly. The usual dose is 1 milligram and is generally considered safe. However, it is sometimes very difficult to differentiate an insulin reaction from *early diabetic coma,* an opposite type of reaction, in which glucagon should not be given.

On occasion, a doctor will give a patient a prescription for glucagon, instruct the parent to buy it, take it to school, and tell the school nurse to give 1 milligram if the child has an insulin reaction. This is totally unwarranted. A school nurse should not give glucagon unless a physician consultant is readily available, there are signed standing orders, and the nurse has demonstrated proficiency in differentiating insulin reaction from diabetic acidosis (early diabetic coma). Even with all of the foregoing criteria, most school nurses should only give a single dose upon direct telephone order from the physician.

Diabetic acidosis refers to a condition that ensues when the blood sugar rises (because of excessive food intake, too little exercise, or not enough insulin) and the child's diabetes begins to go out of control. The early observable symptoms are somewhat similar to those of an insulin reaction; the child is somewhat confused, disoriented, and semiconscious. There are differentiating features, however, as shown in the table on the next page.

Urticaria (hives) at the site of insulin injection is fairly common and usually goes away after the first week or two of therapy.

Lipodystrophy or breakdown of fatty tissue at the injection site occurs very often. The long-term prognosis for complete disappearance of these lumpy, soft skin swellings or depressions is excellent, though sometimes they last two to ten years.

Long-term complications consist of artery and nerve tract changes, which may produce symptoms in the eyes, heart, brain, kidneys, and legs. These changes take twelve to fifteen years or longer to develop and are rarely seen in school-age children.

	Hypoglycemia	Diabetic Acidosis
History	Insufficient food, excess insulin, excess exercise	Lack of insulin, stress, GI upset, febrile illness
Onset	Relatively rapid, one to three hours	Relatively slow, four to ten hours or more
Symptoms	Anxiety, sweating, hunger, headache, blurred vision, twitching	Increased thirst and urination, loss of appetite, nausea, vomiting
Physical Findings	Pale moist skin, full rapid pulse, dilated pupils, rising blood pressure	Red dry skin, soft eyeballs, deep rapid breathing, falling blood pressure
Laboratory Findings	Low blood sugar, sugar-free urine	High blood sugar, high urine sugar

Adapted from *Textbook of Endocrinology,* Williams, R. H. W. B. Saunders Co., Philadelphia, 1981

The school nurse should be aware that most authorities now agree that patients with well-controlled diabetes have a better chance of escaping these serious blood vessel and nerve changes. The nurse's efforts to help the child maintain good control are very worthwhile.

School Relevance and Role of the School Nurse

Diet and Exercise

Diabetic children in school should be under careful control. They should have a regular regime of insulin, diet, and exercise. Any departures from the daily routine should raise a red flag.

The school nurse is the ideal person to correlate all of these activities, especially with the cafeteria manager and the physical education teacher, or the regular teacher in elementary schools with no organized play activities by a special teacher. These staff members need to be briefed by the nurse on their roles and the importance of diet and exercise.

The nurse should maintain frequent contact with the cafeteria manager to keep informed of any missed meals. Likewise, the teacher should be contacted just as frequently to see that the exercise level remains steady. Rainy-day activities need to be preplanned.

Monitoring of Blood and Urine Sugar

Most nurses are already familiar with paper strips to test urine sugar. The school nurse should also learn how to test blood sugar by the finger-prick technique that allows the closer control doctors are recommending. The technique is simple: the finger is pricked and a drop of blood is absorbed onto a special absorbent paper strip; it is washed with water or wiped with cotton (depending on the method), and the color change is compared to a chart. The child's doctor should instruct the school nurse in proper technique, when to test, and any other concern in which the child may need help at school. The school nurse may have to be the one to initiate the partnership by offering assistance to the doctor.

Family and Physician Contact

Since juvenile diabetes is a relatively rare disease, an individual school nurse will rarely have more than two to four children to monitor at any one time. In small schools there may be none.

It is important to arrange telephone contact with more than one family member and with more than one person in the doctor's office. When diabetic children need help, they need it fast. To avoid rushing to a hospital, the school nurse needs a telephone network that is reliable and available all during the school day.

SECTION 12

COMMON CHILDHOOD RASHES

Rashes Associated with Internal Disease
- Nature of the Disorder
- Symptoms and Brief Description

Allergic Rashes
- Nature of the Disorder
  —Causes of Allergic Rashes
  —Types of Allergic Rashes
- Diagnosis
- Treatment
- Role of the School Nurse

Prevention
- Notification of Vulnerable People
- Measles Outbreak Control

RASHES ASSOCIATED WITH INTERNAL DISEASE

Nature of the Disorder

Rashes associated with internal disease include those from red measles (*rubeola*), German measles (*rubella*), chicken pox, and scarlet fever. All of these conditions are contagious. The most contagious are chicken pox and red measles. The most contagious period begins one to three days before the rash appears, continues for one or two days after the rash appears, and then rapidly diminishes even though the rash may remain a day or two longer. See the chart below.

COMPARISON OF FOUR INTERNAL DISEASES

	Days of fever prior to rash	Days rash continues	Days child remains contagious after onset of fever
Red measles	2–3	5–8	4–6
German measles	0–1	1–2	2–4
Chicken pox	0–1	5–10	2–4
Scarlet fever	0–1	2–4	2–4 (if not treated)

There are many other childhood viral infections that cause various types of rashes, but most occur in children below school age. Examples are roseola and fifth disease; all are mildly contagious.

Red measles and German measles are becoming rare because of successful immunization programs.

All of these diseases can vary in severity; the more severe cases last a little longer and remain contagious longer. Contagion does not end abruptly; the child slowly becomes less contagious. Scarlet fever is not contagious after one day of proper treatment, and if untreated, the child usually recovers spontaneously. A small percentage of children become carriers of the germ (streptococcus) while remaining in good health.

Symptoms and Brief Description

Red measles rash begins on the face, moves to the upper chest, stomach, and back, and finally to the arms. It begins as red spots about the size of a match head, and usually the spots run together. No crusts or scabs are formed. The children have red eyes, runny noses, coughs, and high fevers, and they are quite sick.

German measles begins and spreads the same way, but the rash is faint and sparse and in most cases doesn't spread much. The children usually have no symptoms other than low-grade fever and swollen lymph glands behind and below the ears. The diagnosis is often missed.

Chicken pox always begins with a tiny clear vesicle (water blister) that rapidly breaks and forms a loose crust or red scab from scratching and slight bleeding. It usually begins on the arms and legs and spreads to the trunk and face. The rash continues to erupt for two or three days, so one can see all stages of the sores at any one time—pure blisters to loose crusts.

Scarlet fever almost always begins on the face, neck, and upper chest. In more severe cases it then spreads to the trunk and arms. It starts as a diffuse reddish blush, no discrete spots, and the reddish skin feels rough to the touch, almost like gooseflesh. The child may or may not feel sick, depending on the severity of the disease.

Inexperienced observers will often mistake the disease for red measles, a serious mistake because the treatment is completely different. Untreated scarlet fever can result in serious kidney or heart disease. Scarlatina and scarlet fever are exactly the same disease. Doctors occasionally use the name scarlatina for mild cases so as not to alarm patients unduly.

ALLERGIC RASHES

Nature of the Disorder

Allergic rashes are commonly seen. Impetigo and ringworm are discussed in Section 2.

Causes of Allergic Rashes

1. *Contact dermatitis.* The most common is poison ivy or oak, though there are many other plants whose contact can cause a rash in susceptible individuals. Many substances can cause contact dermatitis; fiberglass particles can make anybody's skin itch and cause a temporary rash. Some children develop allergic rashes from wool or animal fur.

2. *Food rashes.* Food allergy is well known, and rashes therefrom can take multiple forms. A physician's skills are required for diagnosis.

3. *Inhalant rashes.* Certain allergic individuals develop rashes from various dusts, pollens, or other substances.

Types of Allergic Rashes

1. *Hives (urticaria).* Hives usually appear as round or oval, pale reddish spots with slightly raised borders. They are usually the size of a dime or a quarter and occasionally come together to form irregular shapes. The spots come and go and reappear, sometimes several times in an hour or two. Occasionally, the eyelids, lips, or other parts of the body will also swell.

2. *Eczema.* This is an allergic rash usually seen in the bends of the elbows, backs of the knee joints, and cheeks. It can, however, appear almost anywhere on the body except the palms and soles. It is rough and scaly and often bleeds from scratching. It is a chronic condition, and most victims have had it a long time.

3. *Miscellaneous allergic rashes.* There are innumerable types of allergic rashes, varying from large red splotches to scaly, pinpoint scabby sores that can spread and join into larger scabs. These rashes can last from a few minutes to many days.

Diagnosis

At times the school nurse or other personnel will be able to identify the condition with certainty; on occasion a visit to the doctor may be necessary. Rashes from completely different causes may look somewhat alike, but a physician can almost always say whether or not the rash is contagious, even when the cause may escape precise identification.

Treatment

While red measles, German measles, and scarlet fever need various treatments, their rash does not itch enough to require treatment. Scarlet fever can usually be completely cured with penicillin and always needs to be treated by a physician.

The rash of chicken pox only needs to be treated to relieve itching. For a small number of itchy pox, plain calamine lotion helps. For itching all over the body, an oatmeal bath is helpful. One cup of oatmeal, cooked until liquid is evaporated, wrapped in cheesecloth, and swirled in a tub of warm water, makes an excellent soaking solution to relieve itching. A baking soda bath also helps. Use one cup of baking soda in a tubful of hot water.

For rashes not associated with internal disease, like those from impetigo, ringworm, scabies, eczema, and hives, many ointments and lotions are available. In some cases oral antihistamines are helpful. These medications should always be prescribed by a physician.

Role of the School Nurse

There are three questions the school nurse should be prepared to answer:

1. Is the condition contagious?
2. Should the child be excluded from school, and, if so, for how long?
3. Is the condition harmful to the fetus of a pregnant woman?

Rashes associated with internal diseases are almost always contagious; the child should be seen by a doctor and not allowed to reenter school until the doctor says he or she is no longer contagious. Impetigo, ringworm, and scabies are also contagious.

Allergic rashes are never contagious. If the child is comfortable, he or she may safely attend school.

Some children with common childhood diseases are excluded from school longer than necessary. (Each nurse should have access to a copy of the publication by the American Academy of Pediatrics entitled *Report of the Committee on Infectious Diseases,* commonly known as the Red Book. It may be obtained by writing to the Academy at: P.O.

Box 927, Elk Grove Village, IL 60009.) Chicken pox and mumps are the two diseases most commonly excluded for too long. Neither ever requires exclusion for more than seven days, unless complications develop.

PREVENTION

Notification of Vulnerable People

We tend to respond to common childhood diseases with indifference, but they are quite threatening to pregnant women and unimmunized (religous and medical exempted) children. It is important that the nurse knows in advance who these vulnerable people are.

Many women like to keep their pregnancy a secret until they begin to show (to make the time seem shorter, to not jeopardize their job opportunities, etc.). This is true for teachers as well. It is important that the nurse tell newly hired staff of childbearing age that her secret will be kept, but she should inform the nurse of any pregnancy when it is discovered. With this knowledge, the nurse can help her to protect the fetus from exposure to contagious children. (See Section 9.)

Measles Outbreak Control

All reports of suspected measles cases should be investigated rapidly. A measles outbreak exists in a community whenever one case of measles is confirmed. Once an outbreak occurs, preventing dissemination of measles depends on promptly vaccinating susceptible persons. Control activities should not be delayed until laboratory results on suspected cases are received. All persons who cannot readily provide proof of immunity should be vaccinated or excluded from the setting (e.g., school). Documentation of vaccination should be considered adequate only if the date of vaccination is provided.

An effective means of terminating school outbreaks and quickly increasing rates of immunization is to exclude all children or adolescents from the outbreak areas who cannot present valid evidence of immunity. Students can be readmitted immediately after vaccination. Experience with outbreak control indicates that almost all students who are excluded from the outbreak area because they lack evidence of immunity to measles quickly comply with requirements and can be readmitted to school. Pupils who have been exempted from measles vaccination because of medical, religious, or other reasons should be excluded until at least 2 weeks after the onset of rash in the last person with measles in the outbreak area.

Morb & Mort Wkly Rpts, 7/10/87

SECTION 13

SCHOOL-RELATED EMOTIONAL/SOCIAL PROBLEMS

Child Abuse
- Classification
- Description of Abusive Families
- Role Reversal
- School Relevance and Role of the School Nurse
- Intervention and Reporting—State Law

Teenage Pregnancy
- Teenage Pregnancy Rate
- Risks for Mother and Baby
- School Programs for Pregnant Girls
- Pregnant Girls Have Unique Educational Needs
- Tips for Management on a Regular School Campus
- Contraception
- School-Based Clinics and Teenage Pregnancy

Suicide
- Nature of the Condition
- Preteen Suicide

- Identifying the Suicidal Students
  —Suicidal Ideas or Comments
  —Suicidal Gestures
  —Suicidal Attempts
- Groups at Risk
  —Previous Suicide Attempters
  —Troubled Teenagers
  —Alcohol and Other Drug Abusers
  —Adolescents with Mental Illness
  —Child Abuse Victims
  —Rigid, Perfectionist Personalities
  —Precipitating Events
- Providing Help for the Student at Risk
  —In the School Nurse's Clinic
  —In the Classroom
  —In the Administrative Office
- School Suicide Prevention Programs
  —Referral of Students
  —Education
- Managing the Aftermath of Completed Suicide
- References

CHILD ABUSE

Cruelty to children has been practiced in many cultures since the beginning of recorded history and is even a part of the early mythology of many ancient peoples. Infanticide, commercial exploitation, and punishment as exorcism of malevolent spirits have all been extensively practiced in "civilized" as well as in "less civilized" societies. The forms of child abuse commonly seen in America and Europe today, however, differ in various important ways from the practices described above.

Investigations into the type of child abuse seen in our society began in the mid-1940s with reports by radiologist John Caffey. He speculated that multiple fractures in infants and young children could have been purposefully inflicted by parents. Other reports in the medical and lay press and the involvement of social service agencies led to federal intervention. Slowly, during the 1950s and 60s, investigations by physicians (led by Drs. Henry and Ruth Kempe of Denver, CO), social workers, and psychologists led to an understanding of the pathologic dynamics and interactions that are so often seen in families in which an abused or battered child is found.

CLASSIFICATIONS

There are four categories of child abuse:

1. Physical abuse
2. Sexual abuse
3. Emotional abuse
4. Child neglect

All four are dealt with by various state laws, and all require reporting to the proper authorities. Definitions vary but are similar in each state. The last two categories—emotional abuse and neglect—are difficult to define, and usually only severe cases are reported.

Description of Abusive Families

It is generally stated that child abuse occurs at all socioeconomic levels of our society. However, all studies of collected data show that more cases occur among the lower classes. There are probably two explanations for this:

1. Most middle- to upper-class individuals utilize private physicians rather than hospital emergency rooms, and therefore cases are less likely to be reported.

2. Poorer parents cannot afford recreation, babysitters, and other means of relieving the stresses associated with child rearing. Also, at lower socioeconomic levels, more youthful marriages, teenage pregnancies, and illegitimate pregnancies occur.

Abusive parents have never learned to ask for help or to trust others. Learning to trust begins in infancy with eye contact, touching and cuddling, and voice communication. By experiencing pain instead of pleasure and not receiving normal developmental stimulation, they grew up to be noncommunicative, nonnurturing adults.

Some children are abused because they do not fulfill parental expectations. A particularly difficult child (excessive infantile colic, squirmy, or hyperactive) is often abused or neglected and becomes the family scapegoat.

Role Reversal

An abused, neglected, and maltreated child is often the victim of an insidious process by which parents expect the child to take on a nurturing role completely and grossly out of keeping with the child's normal developmental abilities. Some mothers, especially teenagers, have babies out of a need for someone to love them, and they expect the child to fulfill that need. Such a young mother who was herself raised in a stressful situation may lack the ability to nurture. She is apt to respond with anger and blame the baby when faced with the difficult realities of child rearing. As the years pass, this child will be expected to provide more and more support and nurture to the parent. The child, completely unable to fill these unrealistic expectations, slowly develops a deep feeling of guilt and may grow to feel that the physical abuse is deserved. Such children become protective of their parents and refuse to divulge information. As adults, they have problems in developing adequate self-esteem. Normally, children are expected to make mistakes; abused children are not allowed to make mistakes and thus develop poor decision-making abilities. They do not learn that they can control their own lives. (It is this feeling of confidence in our own abilities that gives us the ability to control our actions, even though we may not be able to control our feelings. "Getting mad at the baby is OK; hitting it is not.")

School Relevance and Role of the School Nurse

The school nurse can perform a specific role in effectively intervening on behalf of an abused child.

All bruises, burns, or other lesions should be measured, described, and recorded as to size, shape, and location. Photographs are very helpful. Any statements the child makes about the origin of the lesion should be recorded.

If sexual abuse is reported by a child, the person who received this trust should interview the child and record details. However, a physical examination should be done by a doctor, not by the school nurse.

Intervention and Reporting—State Law

Emotional abuse is almost never reported because its definition is so vague. This type of problem can be handled by the school counselor or principal in addition to the nurse. The home problems are usually so severe that not much can be done at school.

Neglect in school-age children should be reported when a parent refuses to seek treatment for a child with an illness that has a real potential for serious complications. Common examples are untreated middle ear infections or serious impetigo.

Failure to bathe, dirty clothes, or other forms of poor personal hygiene, while regrettable, are not grounds for reporting a case of child neglect.

From the above description, it can readily be seen that merely caring for the injuries or neglect that a maltreated child suffers is a shortsighted approach. All fifty state legislatures now have mandatory reporting requirements.

In about thirty-five states, religious groups have obtained exemptions from child abuse reporting requirements, and forty-four states have laws stating that medical treatment by prayer is not a form of abuse or neglect.

Anyone who suspects that a child has been seriously abused is required by law to report the case to the proper authorities. In schools, the teacher or school nurse usually reports suspected cases to the principal, who then makes the official report to the proper social, legal, or medical agency.

School personnel are only required to *report*. The Department of Human Services is required to *investigate*. Occasionally, due to personnel shortages, case workers from DHS ask school personnel to investigate. I usually recommend that school nurses not do this.

The school nurse is in a particularly advantageous position for detecting abused children. Any child who does not engage in normal play, is withdrawn, or assumes a nurturing role inappropriate to his or her age should raise some suspicion. Gentle attempts at conversations may reveal a guarded attitude about parents and home. Such children should be watched, not only for the nurture they need, but also for other more overt signs of abuse or neglect.

Most communities have hot lines for children seeking help. Devise a means for providing the phone number to suspected victims.

Most states are now connected to computer networks that keep track of child-abuse cases nationwide. Since many abusive parents are very mobile and at the same time evasive about the injuries they inflict, this computerized information can be most helpful in deciding if a child injured under suspicious circumstances has previously been reported for suspected child abuse.

The school nurse obviously will have a small role in the actual treatment of injuries or specific guidance and counseling of parents. However, if the nurse has a basic understanding of the pathologic, emotional, and social processes underlying child abuse, a great deal of support can be given to a very needy child, and some guidance can be provided for school officials concerning the medical aspects of the problem.

An excellent small book that offers warm insight into the short- and long-term traumas suffered by an abused child is *Childhood Comes First,* Ray Helfer, M.D., Box 1781, East Lansing, MI 48823.

TEENAGE PREGNANCY

The United States has the highest rate of teenage pregnancy in the developed countries of the world. Each year, about 10 percent of U.S. teens become pregnant and 5 percent give birth. Most of this 5 percent comprises eighteen- and nineteen-year-old women. The chart shown in Figure 13–1 was published by the Alan Guttmacher Institute in 1981, and the situation has not changed much since then.

Teenage Pregnancy Rate

It is evident from Figure 13–1 that the teenage pregnancy rate in the U.S. is higher than all other countries except the Eastern European countries of Czechoslovakia, East Germany, Yugoslavia, Romania, Hungary, and Bulgaria. The U.S. rate is about the same as Italy and Thailand. Japan's rate is one-eighteenth that of the U.S. For the Netherlands and Switzerland the rate is one-fifth, for the U.S.S.R. it is one-third, and for the United Kingdom it is one-half the U.S. rate. The number of very young girls who become pregnant (under fourteen) varies widely from state to state. The table shown in Figure 13–2 was compiled in 1978.

Risks for Mother and Baby

There are no physiological reasons why a sixteen- or seventeen-year-old girl cannot have a healthy baby and remain healthy herself. However, in today's social climate, both mother and baby usually suffer physically, emotionally, developmentally, socially, and economically. The mother is frequently isolated socially, negatively stigmatized, economically disadvantaged, and relegated to federally supported health care. Current research shows that for a baby born to a teenage mother, there is increased risk for:

- low birth weight
- prematurity

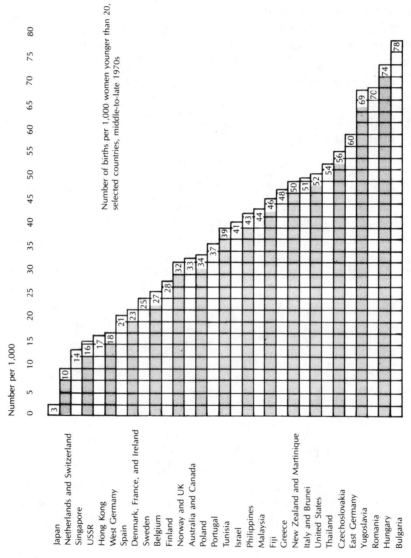

Figure 13–1. Number of births per 1000 women younger than 20: Reprinted with permission from *Teenage Pregnancy: The Problem that Hasn't Gone Away,* Joy G. Dryfoos and Richard Lincoln. Copyright The Alan Guttmacher Institute, 1981.

U.S. total	10,770	Missouri	220
Alabama	410	Montana	10
Alaska	10	Nebraska	30
Arizona	90	Nevada	30
Arkansas	220	New Hampshire	10
California	780	New Jersey	280
Colorado	80	New Mexico	60
Connecticut	90	New York	520
Delaware	60	North Carolina	370
D.C.	70	North Dakota	10
Florida	650	Ohio	380
Georgia	580	Oklahoma	140
Hawaii	20	Oregon	70
Idaho	20	Pennsylvania	380
Illinois	590	Rhode Island	20
Indiana	250	South Carolina	360
Iowa	60	South Dakota	20
Kansas	70	Tennessee	360
Kentucky	260	Texas	1,070
Lousiana	410	Utah	40
Maine	20	Vermont	10
Maryland	240	Virginia	280
Massachusetts	90	Washington	60
Michigan	350	Wisconsin	70
Minnesota	60	Wyoming	10
Mississippi	420		

Figure 13–2. Number of pregnancies to females aged 14 or less: Reprinted with permission from *Factbook on Teenage Pregnancy*, Joy G. Dryfoos and Nancy Bourque-Scholl. Copyright The Alan Guttmacher Institute, 1981.

- birth defects
- child abuse
- learning disability

Among the reasons for these risks are emotional stress, inadequate medical care, poor nutrition, and abuse of alcohol, illegal drugs, caffeine, and tobacco. For the mother there is increased risk for:

- dropping out of school
- complications of pregnancy
- repeat pregnancy
- socioeconomic disruption
- juvenile delinquency

School Programs for Pregnant Girls

The public schools can play an important role in helping pregnant teenagers. Even before she confides in her parents, a girl may approach a school nurse or a counselor to discuss her suspected pregnancy. In most states, a girl has a legal right to privacy, and the parents may not be told without the girl's permission. If the girl refuses permission, there are two important steps that can be taken:

1. Confirm the pregnancy. There are several reliable and inexpensive urine tests to confirm suspected pregnancy. Advising the teen on these products and their use can be valuable.
2. Work with the girl to enlist the help of a legally responsible adult. This may be a parent, other family member, or a social agency.

Many schools will not consider this to be part of their role, but if the school health service department has a medical consultant, arrangements can often be made to confirm the pregnancy if the girl so desires. If the tests are positive, school personnel must then refer the girl to her parents or a special agency.

Some school districts have special classes or special schools for pregnant girls who desire to attend them. An important subject to be taught is normal child development, because over 90 percent of the girls elect to keep their babies. They often expect the baby to love them, not to cry, to be easy to care for, to tolerate being set aside for a while like a play doll, and they have other idealistic and unrealistic expectations. The frustrations and anger that occur when the baby fails to meet these expectations can easily lead to child abuse or neglect. It is well known that young, unmarried mothers are at high risk for physically abusing and neglecting their babies. The girls lack the experience, knowledge, spouse and family support, or the financial resources to get baby-sitters or day care when under stress.

During pregnancy, medical monitoring can be done by a school nurse under the supervision of a physician. In some schools, the doctor visits once or twice a week and is on call for emergencies. Students visit the school nurse's office regularly for medical/nursing evaluation: weight, blood pressure, blood and urine tests, etc. The nurse obtains a comprehensive medical history. During regularly scheduled visits, the nurse discusses nutrition, proper exercise, the meaning of symptoms that occur during pregnancy, normal child development and child abuse, and prevention of future pregnancy. In effect, the nurse becomes the case manager, making home visits, arranging liaison with other physicians and clinics, and helping with bureaucracies (welfare, health departments, etc.).

The health and life-style of the pregnant teenager are closely intertwined, making it necessary for the counselor and the nurse to work as a team, reinforcing each other. Above all, the counselor must be accepting and nonjudgmental. Gossip spreads so fast on school campuses that counselors often choose individual over group sessions. Since pregnant girls are generally socially isolated, group involvement can also be useful if personal confessions are not allowed.

Pregnancy produces a calming and maturing effect on the girls' social behavior. They become less aggressive and boisterous and more conforming to school routine. This persists after the baby is born.

Pregnant Girls Have Unique Educational Needs

1. *Information on what's happening to their bodies.*

2. *Birth control information.* Since 60 percent get pregnant again within five years, this information is very important. Girls believe the wildest rumors about preventing pregnancy, such as jumping up and down so the sperm will get dizzy and not know which way to swim. (See section below.)

3. *Realistic counseling about the father's capabilities.* The father often tells the girl he will take care of all the expenses for the pregnancy and child care. The father sometimes even intends to, but rarely does so. Fathers rarely get involved beyond conception. This difference between promises and actions leaves the girl bewildered and abandoned.

It is better that fathers not be on the same campus. The girls are angry at the boys who get them pregnant and later renege on their promises.

4. *Medical information about pregnancy, delivery, and medications.* Appropriate education relieves anxiety. Body changes from pregnancy, delivery, and nursing can be confusing and upsetting. After delivery, contraceptive pills are blamed for fatigue, hair loss, stomachache, headache, and many other problems. This leads to poor compliance in taking contraceptives. This is frustrating to the nurse, counselor, and parents who fear another pregnancy.

Tips for Management on a Regular School Campus

1. Be patient. These girls are understandably emotionally labile, but respond to caring, understanding, and education.

2. Girls need more water and freedom to go to the bathroom more often. This is particularly evident in the last trimester.

3. They need to get up, stretch and walk around frequently. Some need a small pillow for their back. Others need a footrest or a chair on which to elevate their legs. They ultimately have difficulty squeezing into a school desk; they need a free-moving chair and table.

4. Compromises with the school dress code may be necessary. Feet may swell; necessitating sandals or slippers instead of shoes. In hot weather, loose clothing may be needed. Adding or removing sweaters may occur more often than expected.

5. Assign a nurse, teacher or cafeteria manager to watch the girl's diet. She needs at least two good meals a day. Frequently these are best provided in the school cafeteria, particularly if the teen is socially isolated or not able to afford food at home.

6. Let her participate in all school activities possible that the nurse or doctor permits.

7. Be firm and unyielding in restricting all drugs, alcohol and smoking. With peer group support, there is more chance of abstinence from these chemicals. Research has shown that these substances all have negative consequences on the development, health, and/or birth weight of the infant, as well as on the mother's health.

8. This population of girls seems to have a low tolerance for discomfort. They complain a lot and use the slightest excuse to stay home from school. Be insistent that they come to school. The value of

social and educational opportunities are more important than the comfort of home.

Athletic Guidelines for Pregnant Students in Middle and High Schools

1. Unless a girl has a specific physical problem and a physician's excuse she should participate in some form of physical activity.
2. Emphasize walking as an excellent exercise for pregnant girls, particularly those who were not athletic prior to pregnancy.
3. From the beginning of pregnancy avoid team or individual *competition*. May participate in *recreational* activities: shooting baskets, kicking goals, throwing balls, etc.
4. Because of dangers of hyperthermia and decreased blood flow to the uterus, from the beginning of pregnancy avoid:
   a. Intense exercise in hot, humid weather.
   b. Running or jogging longer than 30 minutes at a time.
   c. Running or jogging for any time period that increases respiratory rate so much that girl cannot engage in ordinary conversation.
5. After the first trimester, no participation in competitive contact sports such as soccer and basketball or competitive sports requiring high intensity exertion, such as track.
6. Provide privacy during shower period.

Contraception

With the easy availability to the girl of contraceptive agents, many assume that sexually active girls will be using some contraceptive method. By age sixteen, 20 percent of female teens have engaged in sexual intercourse. By age nineteen, this rises to 70 percent. Ninety percent of the girls are sexually active prior to marriage. One-fourth of all female teens become pregnant before age nineteen and before marriage. It is estimated that nationally there are 400,000 sexually active girls in the thirteen- and fourteen-year-old age group. Despite these facts, less than 10 percent of sexually active girls use reliable contraceptive methods. Many of the girls who do use methods to prevent pregnancy do not do so consistently or properly.

Some reasons that girls give for not using contraceptives are:

1. Belief that they will not get pregnant. Teenage is a developmental stage where one's limitations are poorly perceived. Teens believe that they totally control their destiny and thus are not aware of the possible consequences of their actions. Boys may drive recklessly and fast, and girls may avoid contraceptives, thinking that accidents and pregnancies won't occur unless they decide that it should. This, of course, produces lots of accidents and pregnancies. It also explains the recklessness with which teens use drugs and alcohol.

2. Willingness to take a chance. Teenage girls do not need to go to Las Vegas to gamble. Some girls see the possibility of pregnancy as a high stakes gamble. The thrill and anxiety which occur make the teen feel "alive" and "excited." This is like drug and alcohol abuse, driving fast, and suicide gestures or attempts. These produce an excitement, like "walking close to the edge of the cliff."

3. Desire to get pregnant. Some girls avoid contraception in the hope that they will get pregnant and thus get a "man" or at least have a baby who they believe will give them the love and caring which they do not find with family or friends. Some girls theorize that "normal" women have babies; if they can then become pregnant, they must be "normal" also, rather than inadequate or alone as they may feel.

4. Passion. Hormones can make passion stronger than conscience. Consequences may not become well focused until after the emotional and sexual activity has subsided. Passion is notoriously difficult for adults to control (as evidenced in music, TV and movies), much less for teens who have less experience or wisdom in these matters.

5. It's not natural. The belief that it is inappropriate to put unnatural substances into one's body leads some girls to avoid various contraceptive measures. Teenagers are often unaware of inconsistencies in this argument; they may use drugs and alcohol but believe that contraception is an unnatural substance.

6. Assumption that boyfriend will use a condom or withdraw early. This is a common but usually unfounded belief. Since boys do not become pregnant, they are traditionally less concerned about condoms or contraception. Passion may play a part here also. Early withdrawal requires cooperation of both partners, cooperation that is rarely available from the boy.

7. Fear friends or family will find out and disapprove. Some girls would rather risk pregnancy than risk a parent finding evidence of contraception. In some groups of girls, contraceptives may lead to social exclusion, whereas in other groups it may be perceived as a status symbol. Some girls have been known to put saccharin tablets in discarded birth control pill containers to get or maintain status in a group.

8. "Cultural" beliefs. Some cultures and individuals see "manhood" evidenced not by adult sexual behavior but by a consequent pregnancy. These male teens may discourage contraception by the girl since it interferes with their perception of their "manhood."

9. Too much bother.

School-Based Clinics and Teenage Pregnancy

In 1965, the Public Health Department of Cambridge, MA located clinics in elementary public schools to deal with common childhood illnesses. They are still functioning and are popular. The first school-based clinics that were developed specifically to reduce the incidence of teenage pregnancy were in St. Paul, MN and Dallas, TX in the late 1960s.

School-based clinics have become controversial because of varying attitudes toward abortion, contraception, and all other aspects of sexuality. Our society has not yet found an effective method to promote premarital sexual abstinence. While thousands of children admit to sexual activity, there is fervent opposition to sex education and school-based clinics, even though the benefits are demonstrable. There are now over 100 school-based clinics operating in the United States, and they all report the following similar findings.

Babies born to mothers who attend schools with a school-based clinic have:

- higher birth weight
- less prematurity
- fewer birth defects
- less child abuse
- fewer school learning and behavior problems when they grow older

Mothers who attend school-based clinics:

- have healthier pregnancies
- have fewer second pregnancies
- finish high school more often (in a well-run program, 75 percent graduate from high school)
- drop out less frequently
- have better job opportunities
- have less juvenile delinquency

Most mainstream health care workers feel that school-based clinics offer an excellent method of reducing the numbers of girls whose lives are adversely affected by an early pregnancy. School-based clinics now offer a wide range of health services, including athletic physical exams, care for common childhood respiratory and gastrointestinal illness, immunizations, and preventive counseling for such problems as drug abuse, suicide, enuresis, and pregnancy.

SUICIDE

Nature of the Condition

Suicide is the successful and intentional taking of one's own life. Because it is so taboo in our society, and for legal, financial, and religious reasons, suicide is often underreported. Well-meaning physicians and coroners often certify a death in suspicious circumstances as accidental rather than suicidal to spare the family additional grief.

The suicide rate in children and adolescents is unquestionably rising. It is now the fourth leading cause of death in the teen years, ranking just behind homicide, cancer, and accidents.

Figure 13–3 demonstrates the rise in suicides during the 1970s in the male population. It also gives an overall rate of suicide of 42 per 100,000 in this age range. It is estimated that 5,000 to 6,000 teens between ages thirteen and eighteen commit suicide each year. This averages out nationally to about one suicide per 4,000 teens per year. Thus, a large high school might expect a suicide each year while smaller high schools could expect one every two or three years. Suicide occurs more often than we would like to think.

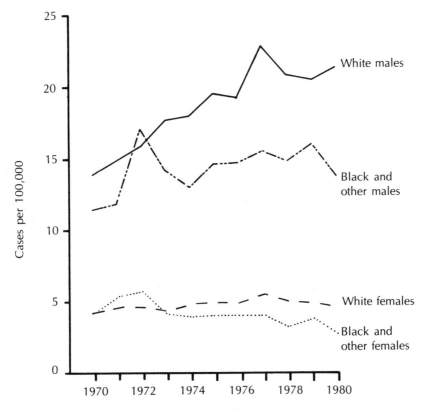

Figure 13–3. Suicide rates for all persons 15–24 years of age, by race and sex—United States, 1970–1980. *Morbidity and Mortality Weekly Reports,* Vol. 36, 1987.

Attempted suicides are much more common; estimates range from 100 to 200 for every successful suicide. Girls make about 90 percent of the attempts, but they are not often successful. Girls usually overdose with pills and can be resuscitated, but in recent years, they have begun to use the same methods as boys. Although boys make fewer attempts, they are more successful because they tend to use more lethal methods, such as guns and hanging, and they seem more intent at being successful. White attempts predominate over Blacks and Hispanics, but the differences are less than in previous years. The incidence is higher in firstborn children.

Increases in suicides have been attributed to many things: increased social and academic pressure on teens leading to increased depression, increased alcohol and drug use, media attention to teen suicide, picturing of and/or glamorization of suicide in TV and movies, less parental supervision, adult role expectations at younger ages, and an increasing number of families where suicide or an attempt has occurred.

Preteen Suicide

As with adolescents, the incidence of suicide and attempted suicide is also rising in children under twelve. These young children come from the same types of homes as suicidal teens and also feel hopeless, helpless, and abandoned.

About the age of ten, children develop more complex thought patterns. Before this time, death is perceived as reversible, much like bad men on TV shows who are killed one week on one show and reappear alive the next week on another. After ten, death can be perceived as irreversible. Suicide and suicide attempts in children younger than ten are frequently imitative of someone who seemed to get attention, publicity or notoriety from the suicide—a relative, a TV character, or a news report. Alarmingly, suicide is often an act which the child believes the parent has requested through comments like "I'd be better off without you" or "You should never have been born." Unfortunately, many parents, in jest or anger, tell their kids these things. Some children then try to please their parents by dying. In children over ten and in teens, suicide may also be a planned solution to escape a dysfunctional family, to join a deceased relative, or to help rid the world of a "bad" or lonely person.

School nurses and teachers need to be alert to the same premonitory signs in younger children as well as in adolescents, especially in children who have "accidentally" ingested poisons. Many studies have shown that over the age of six, true accidental poisoning is rare. The occurrence of repetitive "accidents" may also be an indication of suicidal behavior. Children will give as many hints of suicide as teens, but the hints are generally less obvious. The younger the teen or child is, the easier treatment often is, so early identification is important.

Identifying the Suicidal Student

It is helpful to think of suicidal behavior as a symptom of a medical condition that can be identified, treated, and often cured. A helpful analogy is appendicitis. If properly diagnosed and treated, recovery can be expected. Similarly, suicide is not an isolated event, but rather the last link in a chain of increasingly mortal symptoms of depression. Disregard of the premonitory clues preceding suicide often leads to death; proper diagnosis and treatment can lead to a long and happy life.

Since it is impossible to reverse a completed suicide, attempts to intervene must be made at earlier stages: (1) suicidal ideas or comments, (2) suicidal gestures, and (3) suicidal attempts.

Suicidal Ideas or Comments

Suicidal ideas are the forerunner of suicidal attempts, but they are not easily identified. The teen may (1) be embarrassed and downplay or even lie about the activity, (2) want attention, esteem or notoriety and exaggerate the activity, or (3) lie to protect home situations, parent problems, or friends from exposure. The best plan is to take thoughts about suicide seriously.

Our idiomatic language has many references to death, like "I'm so tired I could die," or "I would rather die than date him/her." These are not considered particularly pathological, but other phrases, like "I am going to die," may be pathological depending on their context. It is important to make early *appropriate* interventions without reacting to every idiomatic expression.

Risk increases in proportion to the amount of suicidal thoughts. Asking how much one thinks of death or suicide can be a good barometer of the need for intervention. Another risk factor is the degree to which a plan has been developed. A teen who thinks of suicide without a means or method planned is at low risk, while someone who plans to take pills or use a gun in a particular setting and at a particular time should be viewed very seriously—even more so if the pills or gun are available.

Suicidal Gestures

Suicide gesture is the term applied to *intentionally* nonlethal attempts. These are often small doses of nonlethal medicines, superficial scratches of the wrist, or other means unlikely to be successful. Suicide gestures are really pleas for help and intervention—the teen can be asking for increased attention of parents or friends, counseling or therapy, release from unbearable situations, or increased adult guidance. Sometimes "suicide gesture" is used in a very pejorative way:

"It was *only* a suicide *gesture!*" This is not only unprofessional and unethical, but dangerous. A suicide gesture is still a cry for help and, thankfully, nonlethal.

Not taking a suicide gesture seriously can lead to escalation to a more lethal level to save self-esteem and to prove that at least they can successfully kill themselves.

Some children engage in suicidal gestures repeatedly. While repeated gestures must be taken seriously, overreaction may provoke more gestures.

Suicidal Attempts

Suicide attempt is the term applied to the legitimate attempt of the teen to harm him- or herself. The attempt may not be successful because of varied reasons: someone unexpected intervenes, the gun misfires, the blood vessel constricts and bleeding stops, a lethal dose was thought to be taken but wasn't, or vomiting occurs. What is clear is that the teen had the *intent* to complete a suicide and took *action* to achieve this goal.

Groups at Risk

Previous Suicide Attempters

Thirty percent of those who successfully complete suicide have made a previous attempt and 70 percent have expressed suicidal thoughts to family or friends. Suicidal thoughts or past attempts are the most reliable guidelines we now have.

Troubled Teenagers

Teenagers who have severe learning problems or conduct disorders (impulsive or aggressive behavior that continually gets them into trouble with family, friends, school, or legal systems) have an increased risk of suicidal behavior.

Depression may be present in these youths, but is generally not apparent; teenagers can be very skillful at hiding their depression. Teenagers who are confused about their sexual identity or who are homosexual clearly are at increased risk.

Alcohol and Other Drug Abusers

For some, substance abuse is only a physical addiction. Others use these substances as a method of coping with interpersonal problems. Still others use drugs for the self-medication of a thought disorder or of depression. Although transient improvement can occur, substance use must increase to maintain the effect, causing physical addiction. Both long-term alcohol use or abuse of other substances can, because of their physiological effects, make a depression worse. Because alcohol and illegal drugs impair judgment, reduce willpower, and eventually deepen depression, they are high-risk factors for suicide. Further, teens may misjudge these drugs and their effects, and take an unintended lethal dose.

Adolescents with Mental Illness

Major depressive disorders such as bipolar affective disorder (manic-depressive illness) are genetically determined mood disorders associated with an abnormality in levels of neurotransmitters within the brain. Onset of these illnesses often occurs in adolescence. Students from families with a history of affective disorders, alcoholism, or suicide (or all three) have a much increased risk of suicide. In some studies, over 90 percent of completed suicides have had a diagnosable mental illness and, of these, 70 percent had sought help prior to the suicide.

Child Abuse Victims

Abused children may think of themselves as bad and responsible for being abused, rather as being the victim. Older children and teens may consider suicide as a response to the feeling of guilt or for having caused their parents so much trouble. Others will consider suicide as a way out of an otherwise hopeless situation. Some feel "You'll be sorry after I'm dead" and see suicide as a means of getting even.

Rigid, Perfectionist Personalities

Adolescents with rigid, perfectionist personality traits have difficulty communicating with peers, experience a great deal of anxiety before tests, and adapt poorly to major life changes. Stress due to either real or perceived parental or school pressure for grade performance may increase their vulnerability. These teens tend not to adjust well to a poor grade, a breakup with a boy- or girlfriend, a move from one school to another, or to intended or unintended embarrassment.

Precipitating Events

A recent loss can precipitate a suicide attempt in a vulnerable youth. This loss may be real, such as the death of a family member or pet, the loss of a job, failing a test, rejection of a boy- or girlfriend, or being arrested. However, the loss may be imagined, with a similar loss of self-esteem, and an increased possibility of suicide.

Clusters of suicides have occurred in communities and even in particular schools. Inappropriate media attention given to a successful suicide can precipitate an attempt in those who may have already been contemplating suicide, or in those teens who are personally insecure and who seek to define themselves by doing what others do. It is important to encourage the media to report the death factually, without discussing means or reasons, and without pictures. The media have an obligation to report these events, and to report them in a way that doesn't encourage other attempts.

Providing Help for the Student at Risk

In the School Nurse's Clinic

Adolescents may present classical symptoms of depression such as mood swings, irritability, appetite and sleep disturbances, and fatigue. More often, however, recurrent headaches, abdominal pain, or other physical complaints may be the symptoms that cause their frequent appearance in the school clinic. Since the school nurse is usually perceived as a helping, nonthreatening person, her sympathetic questioning may well uncover the teen's underlying feelings of sadness, emptiness, lack of interest in usually pleasurable activities, and hopelessness and helplessness for future improvement that are the hallmark of a serious depression.

In the Classroom

Adolescents, rather than presenting classic symptoms of depression, may instead act out through disruptive classroom behavior. Impulsiveness, aggressiveness, apparent boredom, tardiness or truancy, and failing grades in a previously motivated student should be indications for sympathetic questioning, rather than punitive measures. A periodic review of problem students by a team of their teachers might serve to identify students at risk. It should be realized, however, that depression can be well hidden from both family and associates and that suicide is sometimes an impulsive act. Not all cases of suicide can be either predicted or prevented.

Perfectionist, rigid students who have few friends can be gently monitored by teachers and counselors. Befriending them, validating worthwhile personal characteristics, drawing them into group activities, and attempting to diffuse their anxiety about performance can reduce suicide risk. Increasing social involvement of the students also provides a buffer against the loss of a boy- or girlfriend relationship. These teens can be involved in clubs, sports, as teacher aides, etc., if gently, firmly, and personally urged to participate. They are not likely to respond to a general class invitation to participate.

In the Administrative Office

Students at risk for suicide who show up in the principal's office are likely to be those who have been abusing drugs or alcohol, who display aggressive and/or destructive behavior, or who have adjustment problems at home or in school. Some of them may already be known to the juvenile courts in the community. The school may represent the last hope of these students for obtaining adequate help. They should be referred to a mental health center or drug treatment program if there is any suspicion of depression or future suicide.

The threat of school suspension may be used as leverage to induce reluctant students and their parents (who often have a great deal of denial) to accept help from a treatment program, which can be initiated on an outpatient basis with no interruption of school attendance. If hospitalization is necessary to protect the life of the teenager, a phased-in return to school with temporary placement in an alternative class and gradual return to the regular classroom can be coordinated with successful completion of treatment. This implies the need for close cooperation between school authorities and a competent mental health program or drug treatment center designed with the needs of the adolescent in mind. School administrators, counselors, and nurses should be aware of which community programs and private practitioners are well trained and reputable.

School Suicide Prevention Programs

Referral of Students

Each school system should have a mechanism for referral of depressed students or those reported by a peer to have talked of committing suicide. Parents should be urgently invited to come to the school where the concern can be discussed.

Should the school be confronted with a crisis situation where the student makes a suicide attempt on school property, the student should be accompanied to an emergency medical center, usually by ambulance. Reputable hospitals require that a psychiatrist provide an evaluation after the acute medical care has been provided. It is recommended that any attempters be admitted to the hospital until the family situation can be determined and a treatment plan initiated, unless this can be done safely in the emergency room.

While many teens remain suicidal after an attempt and need hospitalization, many do not. The attention, pain, and possibly the treatment itself (forced vomiting, gastric tube, sutures) may alleviate the current suicidal ideas. If the family is responsible and will assure that the teen will get ongoing care, the teen may be safely released. If care is promised, but not provided, the teen will gradually return to suicidal ideas and behavior. School personnel are in a particularly good place to watch for this process and intervene in a timely manner. The school psychologist and guidance counselor may need to provide ongoing counseling if these services are not available. Federal law does require each county to provide for the mental health and mental retardation needs of its citizens. This help is not always adequately publicized.

Education

Each school system should have an ongoing program of education for school faculty and administrators in the behavioral manifestations of depression in adolescents and a knowledge of the suicide risk profile. Procedures for referral should be clearly outlined.

Education should be provided to students each school year concerning symptoms of depression, suicidal behavior, knowledge that help is available through psychotherapy and sometimes the use of antidepressant medications, and the resources available at school and in the community to provide that help. The teacher should explain the necessity of taking seriously and reporting suicidal thoughts expressed by their friends (or themselves) to the school nurse or a sympathetic teacher. The giving away of treasured possessions should be seen as a particularly ominous sign. This kind of education has been shown over and over to decrease attempts rather than encourage them.

Education of parents through newsletters and PTA meetings as to the symptoms of depression, risks of suicide, and necessity of seeking rapid treatment is also important. It should be stressed that any expression of suicidal intent must be taken seriously. The risk involved in keeping a gun in the home (particularly if parents have a family history of depression or suicide) should be pointed out.

Managing the Aftermath of Completed Suicide

Unhappily, in spite of excellent suicide prevention programs, completed suicides still occur. These cases are deeply upsetting for students and teachers alike. The announcement of the death is best made in individual classrooms by teachers or guidance counselors who knew the student rather than in a special assembly or over the public address system. Care should be taken to downplay the drama of the event. Counseling, both immediate and long-term, should be offered to students by guidance counselors and those school psychologists who know the students best. These are usually better accepted by students than having a team of outside professionals come into the school; outside professionals are best reserved to educate teachers and guidance counselors in handling such a situation.

Students who are contemplating a similar suicide may display unusual interest in the details of the death of the student, may make more than one visit to the funeral home or grave site, and may seem obsessed with the event even though the student who committed suicide may not have been a close friend. Observance of such behavior by parents or teachers should initiate referral to the counselor or school nurse.

References

Beck, A. T., R. A. Steer, M. Kovacs, and E. Garrison. "Hopelessness and Eventual Suicide: A 10-Year Prospective Study of Patients Hospitalized with Suicide Ideation," *American Journal of Psychiatry*, May 1985, 142 (5): 559–563.

Gould, M. S., and D. Shaffer. "The Impact of Suicide in Television Movies: Evidence of Imitation," *New England Journal of Medicine,* 1986: 680–694.

Mental Health, United States, NIH Division Biometry and Epidemiology, 5600 Fishers Lane, Rockville, Maryland 20857, 1985.

Robins, Eli, *The Final Months: A Study of the Lives of 134 Persons Who Committed Suicide.* New York: Oxford University Press, 1981.

Ross, C. P. "Mobilizing Schools for Suicide Prevention," *Suicide and Life Threatening Behavior,* 1980, 10 (4): 239–243.

Shaffer, David. Paper on suicide and depression in children and adolescents (NIMH study), *Adolescent Study,* 1985.

SECTION 14

BEHAVIOR DISORDERS

School Refusal and Phobia
- Nature of the Condition
  —School Refusal
  —School Phobia
- Treatment

Speech Disorders
- Stuttering
- Articulation Disorders
- Elective Mutism

Enuresis
- Nature of the Condition
- School Relevance and Management

Encopresis
- Nature of the Condition
- School Relevance and Management

Childhood Depression
- Nature of the Condition
- Classification
- Symptoms
  —Overt
  —Masked
- Treatment and School Relevance

Autism
- Nature of the Condition
- Symptoms
- Relationship to Mental Retardation
- Organic Brain Damage
- Prognosis
- Treatment and School Relevance
- Five Common Myths Concerning Autism

Anorexia Nervosa
- Nature of the Condition
- Symptoms
- Psychological Profile
- Diagnosis
- Treatment
- Prognosis
- School Relevance and Role of the School Nurse

Bulimia

Sleeping in School
- Nature of the Condition
- Diagnosis
  - —Insufficient Sleep
  - —Emotional Reaction
  - —Narcolepsy
- Treatment
- Role of the School Nurse

SCHOOL REFUSAL AND PHOBIA

Nature of the Condition

Many children harbor unexpressed as well as overt fears about school. When the fear is so great that it causes the child to avoid going to school, it is necessary to determine the cause of the extended absence because the management of each case is highly specific.

School Refusal

A child may refuse to go to school for fear of a bully; another may feel unprepared for a test. An older child may simply regard school as irrelevant to his or her entire value system and future life.

Some children instead of being afraid of the school setting, may be fearful of leaving home because of:

1. Jealousy of a younger sibling at home
2. Parental conflict, causing fear for the mother's safety in the child's absence
3. Fear of abandonment, especially when one parent has recently left
4. A recent death in the family, since the child may equate death with going away

Though these children need to learn more productive coping skills, this type of reaction pattern is not altogether abnormal. These reasons for truancy and absenteeism are not considered phobic.

School Phobia

Mental health specialists usually reserve the diagnosis of school phobia for those cases in which there is an abnormally close relationship between the child and the mother; when apart they both suffer separation anxiety. Therefore, limiting management to the child always fails; the parents must be equally involved.

School phobia occurs more often in a large family with relatively few outside contacts, where many relatives live in close physical proximity, and the child's parents are often closely involved with the grandparents. It is not the size of the family that is a factor; it is the isolation of that family group, extended or nuclear, from the community.

A school-phobic child who is forced to attend school can be expected to have many somatic complaints such as headache, stomachache, and other body aches. Other symptoms are crying, whining, sulking, and running away from school.

Treatment

Management of a school-refusing or school-phobic student requires cooperation from parents, the school nurse, teacher, counselor, therapist, and most important, the school principal. The principal's support will determine the effectiveness of the school's role in therapy. Insight into the psychodynamics of the family's cultural and religious values will help the principal help the family.

School phobia should be seen as a potentially serious condition, having ramifications beyond school. It affects a child's social relations as well as academic performance. If the family is left to its own devices, the child will rarely return to school.

All therapy is based on returning the child to school as soon as possible. All studies have shown that the longer a child remains out of school after the onset of symptoms, the longer treatment is necessary, sometimes taking months or years. Suggestions which may be useful in management include the following:

1. The person most likely to be successful in convincing the mother to initiate treatment is often the school person whom the child knows (teacher, nurse, counselor, or principal.

2. These mothers are particularly in need of an understanding and reassuring principal who will not become defensive. She will grasp at any justification to keep a phobic child at home—fear of failure, peer ridicule, or a strict teacher are her typical rationalizations for keeping the child at home.

3. The object is to return the child to school. Family counselling may be necessary before this can be initiated. School phobia is more difficult to manage in older children.

4. A suggested technique for reducing anxiety is to have the mother and child visit the school briefly, perhaps walk down the hall together and return home. Insist that the child spend a little more time each visit—include a friendly greeting from the librarian and the school nurse on a second visit.

5. Adults must be alert to the nurturing needs of these frightened children, especially not allowing peers to victimize them.

SPEECH DISORDERS

Stuttering

Children respond to their mothers' voices in the early weeks and months of life, long before they acquire an understanding of symbolic language. Receptive language ability continues to exceed expressive language ability throughout life.

Between the ages of two and four years, children have an urgent need to express themselves before they have developed the language fluency to do so. This is often called the period of dysfluency and is characterized by frequent syllabic repetition. If adults express concern about this normal phenomenon, the child is made to feel inadequate about his or her speech, causing self-conscious focus on the mechanics of speaking. This can impair the normal development of fluency and cause stuttering.

Of course, many other factors can also cause stuttering. Children who begin to stutter at age six or seven need a different therapeutic approach from that of a three- or four-year-old. The school nurse should suggest that the older child be seen by the school psychologist as well as the speech pathologist.

Articulation Disorders

Errors of articulation may consist of distortions, substitutions, omissions, or lisps. Occasionally, a structural abnormality of the mouth, tongue, or palate can cause difficulty; often there is no demonstrable pathology. When remediation is necessary, the child must be referred to the speech pathologist. However, there are some children whose minor articulation imperfections are barely noticeable and who are always understood.

In all probability, these children will never be handicapped by their slight lisps or occasional consonant omissions. Since referral to a speech pathologist is often stigmatizing, the school nurse can ask the speech pathologist to make a casual classroom visit for verification of the need for speech therapy.

Elective Mutism

A child who is shy by nature and speaks very little at home or at play may react to extra stress by the development of elective mutism (sometimes called selective mutism). This child is not being willful or obstinate; the inability to speak is an adaptive reaction to stress.

This rare condition, when seen, often begins at school in the elementary grades. The parents usually state that the child does speak when not in school. Often one of the parents also has a shy, retiring disposition.

Elective mutism usually causes great consternation at school; teacher, counselor, and principal vie with one another to see who can get the child to talk. This approach, of course, is counterproductive because the extra attention only serves to reinforce the gain that the child receives from remaining mute. Successful therapy requires complete cooperation from all school personnel and should always be supervised by a psychologist skilled in behavior management techniques.

If a child is placed in an institution, rapid results may be achieved because of the strict control available; however, relapses are common with return to the previous environment. The goal of therapy is not merely to have the child say some words, but to react to stressful situations in a more normal manner.

Case histories following children with elective mutism over a long period of time report eventual normal speech. However, 5 to 25 percent remain very poor communicators. How much of a handicap this is in later life depends on the individual's vocational choice and life style.

ENURESIS

Nature of the Condition

Urinary incontinence with soiling of clothes can occur during the day or night. Though some children are toilet trained by age three, so many children have frequent accidents up to age five that it can hardly be considered abnormal. Between the ages of three and six, whether it is considered abnormal or not depends a great deal on parental expectations. In some families, there is a great deal of parental pressure for early toilet training. If the child, for whatever reason, is not constitutionally ready, or if he or she subconsciously rebels, this parental attitude is apt to cause the child to be labeled as *enuretic*. The label itself can contribute to prolonged wetting. Another child with this same problem in a relaxed household might well become completely toilet trained, day and night, by age four or five. Most pediatricians do not consider bed wetting sufficiently abnormal to require treatment before the child is six years old.

While an occasional child with enuresis will be found to have some infection or abnormality of the urinary tract, the large majority will not. The causes of nonorganic enuresis at school are legion. Examples are: too early and too demanding toilet training, and fear of going to the school rest room.

School Relevance and Management

The following plan is by Donna Von Merz, a San Antonio school nurse who, on her own initiative, developed an individual plan for each enuretic student on her campus:

> "Kindergarten and first grade children are often afraid of the large public bathroom in public schools. Debbie had never had 'accidents' at home. She was afraid of two things: the powerful flushing of the school toilets, which was so much louder than the one at home, and at home her mother allowed her to leave the bathroom door open, while at school the other girls always closed it.

"This is the schedule I worked out for Debbie. Just before class time, at about 7:50 a.m. Debbie came to the health room (clinic) to urinate in the clinic toilet. For the first week I had to get her; after that, she came on her own. At about 9:30, 11:00 and 12:30, she came again to the clinic to urinate. At 2:00 she also came and (luckily, on her own) also had a bowel movement.

"After seven to ten days, I began to accompany her to the main restroom and wait for her to finish. I did this three or four times and then she was willing to go by herself. From that time on, she has remained dry. The whole process took about four weeks."

This nurse also emphasizes the importance of keeping spare clothes at school so that accidents can be handled privately and unobtrusively. Also, holidays or prolonged absences may be followed by regression, so a little "preventive action" is wise *before* accidents reoccur.

This is an individual and holistic approach to a problem that can often be easily managed, but if mismanaged, may develop into a major school malfunction.

It has always been traditional to rule out urinary tract infection in children with enuresis. One can't argue with this advice; however, it costs about $25 to visit the doctor's office plus $15 each for two or three urinalyses. Also, it usually means a day off from work for the parent. While my pediatric instincts recommend urinalyses, I see nothing wrong with a school nurse using the above approach for a child with a history like Debbie's—no wet pants at home and no evidence of ill health.

Almost all kindergarten and first grade teachers know that many children have "accidents," and they try to protect these children from embarrassment. By the second or third grade, however, repeated urinary soiling is rare enough to be considered abnormal, and the child should be referred to a physician.

In some cases, the amount of urine expelled is so small that it can be safely ignored if it creates no disturbance.

If the teacher feels confident that the child is not using the symptom for some secondary gain, a discreet method of having the child go to the rest room once or twice a day can be arranged.

When a child is noticeably wet and smells of urine almost every day, management should be the same as for overflow incontinence of the bladder. This happens regularly in certain diseases of the lower spinal cord such as spina bifida. (See Section 17.) The parents should provide extra clothes so the child can be helped to change clothes privately.

ENCOPRESIS

Nature of the Condition

Habitual fecal soiling occurring past the ages of five to seven is known as *encopresis*. Not only are the causes more complicated than those of enuresis, but, because of the odor, more adverse social consequences are suffered.

As in children with enuresis, children with encopresis are rarely found to have organic disease or abnormality requiring surgery or specific medication. A notable exception is chronic and severe constipation. Normally, the rectum slowly fills and, at a certain point of stretch, the nerve endings send the proper message to the brain so that the individual has a normal bowel movement. If for some reason the rectum is not evacuated at that time, the urge eventually goes away until a later time. Children who are sufficiently constipated lose the urge altogether and develop a fecal impaction, a large hard mass of stool that gathers at the lower rectum and causes obstruction. The stool above the impaction then liquefies and leaks around the impaction. (See Figure 14–1.)

Though the child is completely unaware that this is happening, the underwear is constantly soiled and the fecal odor invites derision from classmates.

Fecal soiling may also occur simply because the child will not take the time to go to the bathroom. In this case, there will be a good-sized mass of stool in the pants, not the lesser amount that is seen in the overflow incontinence just described.

School Relevance and Management

Treatment is administered by a physician. A fecal impaction is easily diagnosed by a digital rectal examination. It can be removed by a gentle water or mineral oil enema, repeated two to three times if

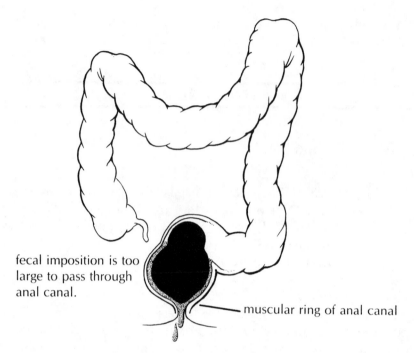

fecal imposition is too
large to pass through
anal canal.

muscular ring of anal canal

Figure 14–1. Fecal Impaction

necessary, plus mineral oil given by mouth. Each child's oral dose of
mineral oil is different; it should be given every night or two in an
amount sufficient to cause a full-sized soft stool each day but not
enough to cause leaks and stained pants. For children who dislike plain
mineral oil, there are several emulsified flavored products available.
After sufficient time, usually three to six months, the rectum regains its
tone and rhythmicity, and bowel movements can occur normally
without mineral oil.

Classroom management is similar to that of the severe enuretic.
An extra set of clothes should always be on hand, and the nurse should
enlist the aid of the teacher, counselor, and principal to help the child
get to the bathroom with as little humiliation as possible.

Children who do not have a fecal impaction yet do have a problem
with soiling, may be helped by psychological counseling or behavior
management techniques.

CHILDHOOD DEPRESSION

Nature of the Condition

All normal individuals, child and adult, feel depressed at various times in their lives. However, when mental health specialists speak of *depression*, they don't mean temporarily feeling down; they mean a distinct disease entity that strongly affects the total personality. Depression usually lasts several months or years and often requires specific medical or psychiatric treatment such as psychotherapy or psychoactive medication. There is no question that depression is one of the most common psychiatric disorders in adults. It also occurs with less frequency in children.

Classification

1. *Endogenous depression* implies that the patient has an innate or inborn psychological weakness that predisposes him or her to depression.
2. *Reactive depression* is thought to be caused by adverse environmental or situational circumstances. In school children, a suspected cause is continued classroom failure and repeated loss in most of the everyday life struggles that all children face.

Symptoms

Overt

1. Feelings of boredom, helplessness, or hopelessness
2. Loneliness, isolation, or withdrawal
3. Feelings of sadness
4. Diminished enthusiasm and physical activity
5. Self-deprecatory statements
6. Suicidal ideas, expressions, or actual attempts

Masked

The masked symptoms are those compensatory or coping mechanisms the depressed child develops to protect his or her self-esteem:

> The wish to avoid sadness and humiliation is a powerful motivating force and a major determinant of behavior for all school-age children. If a child cannot measure up to expected school performance, he [or she] often will react with some form of socially maladaptive behavior to save face. Children are forced to participate in activities that expose them to failure and ridicule. Many adults also are engaged in a constant effort to avoid humiliation, but for them the task is an easier one. If they can't dance, they don't go to dances! If they are not good at reading, they can go to movies! Children, however, are required to pursue activities that display weaknesses likely to lead to humiliation. (Adapted from Levine, Brooks, and Shonkoff's *A Pediatric Approach to Learning Disorders* New York: John Wiley & Sons, 1980.)

Depression can be expressed by these masked symptoms:

1. Headaches, stomachaches, or other body complaints.
2. Silliness and clowning
3. Aggression, fighting, and rebelliousness
4. Poor school performance
5. Physical tiredness (often in adolescents)
6. Drug use in adolescents. If an adolescent does not know how to communicate fear or anger, the use of drugs removes the emotional discomfort.

Long term studies of large groups of children at various ages have been done to determine the frequency of symptoms of masked depression in a healthy population, since normal children have these symptoms at various times in their lives. One study of seventh and eighth grade children (Kovacs and Beck) showed that 33 percent were depressed to a degree labeled moderately severe. Such a high incidence rate casts doubt on the validity of the diagnosis, especially since all of the "normal" children were performing well in school. This and other studies have led researchers to the following conclusion:

> The concept of a syndrome of masked childhood depression is as yet unsubstantiated and . . . a diagnosis of this condition in children would appear to be premature and treatment unwar-

ranted. The possibility of producing iatrogenic (doctor-induced) effects on the child, the risk of masking other problems, and the unknown effects on the parents underscore the need for rigorous research of this question.
(Lefkowitz and Buron, 1978)

Over the last three years, the existence of "masked depression" has been thought to be less likely.

Treatment and School Relevance

Management of the so-called depressed child cannot be generalized; treatment is aimed at the symptoms. However, school nurses and teachers can be guided by certain principals:

1. Never try to manage a depressed child without professional consultation from a psychologist, psychiatrist, or family doctor. Involve the counselor, principal, and parents as much as possible.

2. Depressed children are moody and suffer from low self-esteem. Though it is easier for a teacher to deal with a sad, quiet six-year-old than an angry, belligerent thirteen-year-old, both need skilled intervention.

3. It will be impossible for a classroom teacher to take time to meet all the needs of a depressed child. It is important, however, to have some insight into the underlying problems so as not to unknowingly embarrass the child and perhaps provoke further maladaptive behavior.

4. Maladaptive behavior must not be condoned. While one cannot be overly strict in every detail, it is important for such children to know that the teacher is aware of what they are doing. Aggression, giving up too easily, poor school performance, and so on, should be confronted confidentially and directly, not glossed over.

5. Consistent, sustained academic achievement is not a priority for depressed children. If they can be taught to sublimate their aggression, perform easy-to-complete tasks, relate to peers, and assume some age-appropriate responsibilities, their achievement and self-concept will also improve.

6. Drug treatment of childhood depression with adult-type, mood-elevating medication is quite controversial at this time. Some children do seem to benefit from its use, however, and a school nurse

can make a real contribution to the child's therapy by observing and reporting changes in behavior. Tofranil and Elavil are the medications most commonly used. They are not approved by the FDA for children under twelve. They have the potential of causing adverse cardiac and bone-marrow reactions. Also, there is strong evidence for a placebo effect.

AUTISM

Nature of the Condition

Autism is sometimes thought of as infantile or early childhood schizophrenia, but the differences between the autistic child and the preteen or adolescent schizophrenic are so great that the prevailing consensus is that they are separate and distinct conditions.

Originally it was believed that autism in children was largely caused by a lack of nurturing and improper parenting; it was thought to exist in the children of cold and aloof parents. However, it is now fairly universally agreed that autism is an organic developmental disability whose cause is not related to parental management.

Autism is a very strange disorder. It is relatively rare, and some school nurses, especially in the upper grades, have never seen a case. However, it would be beneficial to visit a facility for autistic children or to see a documentary film showing such children at various ages and activities.

Symptoms

1. *Aloneness.* Autistic children truly live in a world of their own. They relate to people as they relate to a table. Occasionally the child will respond to speech, but erratically, seldom, and often inappropriately. Occasionally they will speak, but with little relationship to what is happening or what they want.

2. *Onset at an early age.* Symptoms always appear before three years of age. Occasionally, with hindsight, parents can recall that during infancy their baby would not cuddle or snuggle. As toddlers, they did not follow their parents or go to them for comfort.

3. *Delayed and deviant language development.* Fully 50 percent never gain useful speech, and those who do often use it in an abnormal fashion. There is persistent *echolalia* (echoing the words of others) of words and phrases and error in choice of pronoun (I–you). Speech is used in a noncommunicative manner—it lacks a give-and-take quality. Only the present exists; what happened earlier is never mentioned. The precursors of oral language, such as "pat-a-cake" or "bye-bye," don't develop. Speech onset is late and comprehension is very poor. There is a lack of appropriate gesture—instead of pointing with the finger, the whole hand is used; if the child wants an object, he or she will take an adult's hand and lead the adult to it rather than ask for it. Simple spoken commands by a parent or teacher require accompanying gestures for complete understanding.

4. *Grossly impaired social development with specific characteristics.*

a. Quality of aloneness described above.

b. A compulsive insistence on sameness, with resistance to change. Requires same object at all times. Older children become obsessed with bus routes, colors, numbers, and so on.

c. Ritualistic behavior such as touching.

d. Lack of cooperative group play. No imaginative games. Much stereotyped and repetitive behavior.

e. No friends.

f. Lack of empathy or ability to perceive feelings of others. Often saying or doing things that are socially inappropriate.

g. Eye contact deficient and abnormal. "Even when he looks at me, he doesn't seem to be seeing me."

h. Occasional exceptional rote memory.

Relationship to Mental Retardation

Skillful testing has revealed that autistic children vary greatly in their intellectual capacity and that IQ scores are good predictors of educational attainments. Also, it appears that IQ scores remain stable over long periods of time. Thus, it is felt that an autistic child with a very low IQ score is just as retarded as a nonautistic child with a very low IQ score. Autism and mental retardation may coexist.

Most autistic children have a normal physical appearance, but those with concomitant mental retardation may have the facial features commonly seen in nonautistic retarded children. Also, autistics with a phenomenal rote memory will usually have a high IQ. These children are sometimes called "idiot savant," or more recently "autistic savant."

Those with lower IQ scores are apt to be less socially competent; they are prone to exhibit more bizarre behavior (inflict self-injury, smell other people, etc.).

Organic Brain Damage

As yet, no specific, localized brain damage that is consistent for all autistics has been found. A sizeable proportion of autistic children develop neurologic abnormalities such as epilepsy in later life, especially those with lower IQ scores.

As stated earlier, the consensus is that there is some undetected anatomical or chemical brain abnormality. Since the first edition of this book, several reliable studies have confirmed this consensus.

Prognosis

Much depends on the intellectual level. If the IQ score is over 70, about 75 percent gain competency in basic arithmetic skills and go on to more education or find paid employment. If the IQ score is below 70, the figure is only 20 percent.

The overall prognosis for the autistic child is generally unfavorable; most eventually reside in institutions. To keep an older autistic child at home requires special physical and caretaking facilities that most parents do not have. An autistic child with superior intellectual capacity will be educable, and extra efforts in his or her behalf are well worth the time and energy required.

Treatment and School Relevance

As can be imagined, many and various treatments, rational and irrational, have been tried. None has succeeded with any consistency. Occasionally a case is reported to have improved with vitamins, minerals, manipulations, and so on. Naturally, a parent will not stop using any irrational treatment if it appears to be helping, so unless it is actually harmful it is usually best to adopt a wait-and-see attitude.

The only "therapy" that consistently yields good results is proper behavior modification, often requiring strong aversive methods. This type of therapy only modifies symptoms but is quite effective and especially necessary to control self-destructive actions such as severe head banging or biting.

Classroom management is extremely difficult. Most often a special facility is required, but if a teacher has an autistic child in class, that teacher has every right to demand expert professional assistance and consultation. Through medical or psychiatric contacts, the school nurse can help in this liaison.

Fenfluramine is a newer drug that is now used to treat autism. There are conflicting reports as to its effectiveness. Some experts say it is ineffective and it may have serious adverse side effects.

There is currently wide interest in a behavioral method which recommends that the patient receive strong body hugging. Time and controlled studies will be necessary to assess the effectiveness of this therapy.

Parents of these children are equally in need of help. Their greatest need is to be able to get away at frequent intervals. In many large cities, respite care facilities are available, but if not, private-duty nurses or tranquilizing medications may be necessary. Parent self-help organizations are very helpful, and the school nurse can help the parents locate them. Since the passage of P.L. 94-142, more school districts throughout the United States have developed special facilities for autistic children.

FIVE COMMON MYTHS CONCERNING AUTISM

False	True
Autism is an emotional disorder.	It is organic.
Children grow up to be schizophrenic adults.	Genetically different from schizophrenia. Adults usually are retarded.
Children do not look retarded, and have normal cognitive potential.	Normal intelligence is very rare. Very few ever handle college.
"Idiots savant" understand what they repeat, say, or draw.	They have rote abilities without understanding what they are repeating, neither verbally nor with a pencil or crayon.
Untestable or very difficult to test	Not if test is geared low enough.

From J. M. Farber et al., *Clinical Pediatrics*, April 1984, page 189. Used with permission.

ANOREXIA NERVOSA

Nature of the Condition

Anorexia nervosa can be described as a relentless pursuit of
excessive thinness. It is not a dislike of food, simply a pathological
desire to be always thinner and thinner. Patients are obsessed with
food, they enjoy preparing it for others, and they frequently work at
food-related jobs, such as waiting on tables. They collect large numbers
of diet cookbooks. When they do eat, they often cut their food up into
tiny pieces and chew each one slowly so that a meal may last an
inordinately long time.

At first, the dieting is mild and intentional, and the patient
receives approval. However, the sinister nature of the disease slowly
manifests itself, and losing weight becomes an obsession; no matter
how thin they become, the patients always want to be thinner. Finally,
after sufficient weight loss, symptoms of starvation such as debility,
fatigue, and clouding of consciousness begin to take their toll.

Symptoms

Ninety to 95 percent of patients are girls between fifteen and
nineteen years of age who were never overweight to any remarkable
degree. The condition sometimes begins as young as eleven years and
as old as forty years. By the time the patients come to medical attention
they are shockingly thin. As long ago as 1689, a Dr. Richard Martin
described a patient: "I do not remember that I did ever in all my
practice see one . . . so much wasted . . . (like a skeleton only clad with
skin) yet there was no fever but on the contrary a coldness of the whole
body."

There is always intense family involvement and interaction. At
first the parents merely tell their daughter that she is thin enough, but
they soon discover that she wants to be forever thinner. Sometimes
they force the child to eat but this often leads to induced vomiting,
either openly or secretly. The disease may have existed for quite some
time before the parents are even aware of it because at this age parents
don't see their children undressed, and the facial fat pads don't
disappear until late in the process of starvation.

The daily calorie intake becomes an obsession. A girl who has put herself on a diet of 800 calories per day (already dangerously low) may cut it down to 400 calories per day "just to be sure."

Vomiting, spontaneously or with the help of a finger or spoon down the throat, is a dangerous complication. Some anorexic patients develop bulimia and vomit after a binge of rapid, excessive eating.

Excessive laxatives and diuretics may be used along with induced vomiting. The laxative excess causes burning and pain in the stomach with intestinal cramps. In addition, there is a dangerous loss of minerals, particularly sodium and potassium. Patients who vomit and overuse laxatives and diuretics are in particular danger, and it is in this group of young girls that fatalities may occur.

Exercise excess as a method of burning up calories often occurs in the form of bicycling, running, swimming, and calisthenics. As patients get thinner, they exercise even more.

Mirror gazing occasionally occurs. Patients will stand nude in front of a mirror for long periods of time, never recognizing or acknowledging their thinness, though they may be a mere "bag of bones." This is considered a poor prognostic sign.

Amenorrhea (cessation of menstruation) eventually occurs in all anorexic girls, and in about half of the cases, the menstrual periods stop at about the same time as the dieting begins. It is known that prolonged starvation causes cessation of menstruation (as in women in prisoner-of-war camps); therefore, it was first thought that the amenorrhea of anorexia nervosa was caused only by the severe weight loss. Since about half of the patients stop menstruating before they lose any appreciable weight, it is postulated that there may be some primary disturbance in the hypothalamus, a part of the brain that controls appetite and also, to some extent, menstruation. The significance of this dilemma remains undecided.

Stealing is seen in some patients, usually food at first in binge eaters, and then money to buy food. Later they may begin stealing trinkets or jewelry to wear for adornment. The stealing has a compulsive quality to it and usually stops after successful treatment of the anorexia nervosa.

The typical patient comes to the doctor about one to two years after dieting, vomiting or purging, and beginning of excessive exercises and family disruption. They usually have lost about 20 to 40 percent of their ideal body weight and are very emaciated, but they do not think of themselves as being excessively thin. They have a characteristic life style that derives satisfaction only from the denial of calories and refusal of outside help from parents, physicians, or other health professionals. When they do finally go to the doctor, they reject any suggestions that they should increase their caloric intake.

Psychological Profile

Girls with anorexia nervosa are usually of a compulsive nature. They maintain a neat appearance and are concerned about proper clothing and grooming. They usually get good grades in school, often higher than one would expect from the IQ tests. However, they seem to be joyless individuals and derive little satisfaction from their good grades. They often have strong feelings of helplessness and unworthiness with a paralyzing sense of ineffectiveness. Parents often describe their daughter as the perfect child. Adjectives commonly used to describe her are cooperative, obedient, intelligent, thoughtful, considerate, and even-tempered; "she's the last one who would have caused trouble."

Diagnosis

The diagnostic criteria are as follows:

1. Fear of obesity becoming worse as the patient gets thinner
2. Disturbance of body image; feeling fat even when thin
3. Loss of at least 25 percent of original body weight
4. Refusal to maintain body weight over minimum normal weight for age and height
5. No other physical or mental illness that accounts for weight loss
6. Amenorrhea (eventually seen in almost all patients)

Treatment

The earlier the disease is recognized and treatment is begun, the better are the chances for cure. Most established cases require a period of separation from the family, usually in a hospital. Treatment must be both psychologically and medically oriented. Strict behavior modification with clearly defined goals (such as one to three pounds of weight gain per week) is the method usually employed today. The diet must be carefully selected so it will be acceptable to the patient and will also restore minerals, vitamins, and all other nutrients. Only rare severe cases require tube feeding and intravenous feeding.

Prognosis

Considering all types of cases from mild to severe, the long-term outlook is not particularly favorable. The usual figures quoted are about as follows:

Good outcome—40 percent
Intermediate outcome—30 percent
Poor outcome—25 percent

The mortality rate is 2 to 5 percent. Death is usually caused by an infection (such as pneumonia) at a time when all of the body resources are so depleted that all resistance is gone and no antibodies can be manufactured to fight the disease.

In the 70 percent of patients who recover, most remain preoccupied with diet and weight for many years. Recurrences are common. Only about 20 to 25 percent of all cases return to perfectly normal health.

A poor prognosis can be guessed at if the following factors exist: long duration, lower weight at beginning of treatment, unsuccessful past treatment, vomiting, and excess use of laxatives and diuretics.

School Relevance and Role of the School Nurse

Since most cases begin in girls of high school age, school personnel can play a large part in early diagnosis and can also assist in treatment. Those most involved will be the school nurse, the counselor or principal, and the physical education teacher.

The school nurse is in a position to integrate the efforts of the parents, school personnel, and physican. Any girl who shows the two most outstanding symptoms—sadness or solitude and weight loss—should be watched for a time to see if initial suspicions are confirmed.

The physical education teacher should be consulted to see if the girl resists "suiting up" and, if she does, whether she is unusually thin. If necessary, the student can be asked to come to the clinic weekly or monthly to be weighed. Since this is usually a growth period, any sustained weight loss should raise a red flag and the other symptoms can be looked for.

Parents usually discover the disease quite late in its course, and since the prognosis is better with an early diagnosis school personnel can play a key role. All that is required is an awareness of the disease and a relatively high index of suspicion.

Once the diagnosis is established, the school nurse can integrate and support the parents' and physician's efforts. The counselor and physical education teacher can be enlisted to form a team that is actively supportive and thus assist in producing a favorable outcome.

There are two concrete steps the school nurse can take to help in therapy:

1. Weekly or monthly weighing with support and encouragement
2. Letting the patient use the school clinic as a refuge (Girls with anorexia, being somewhat depressed and feeling helpless, need support from as many sources as possible.)

BULIMIA

Pure *bulimia* consists of episodic and uncontrollable urges to eat excessively and an inability to stop. These episodes are called binges. The food chosen is usually sweet, highly caloric, and capable of being eaten rapidly with little chewing. Binge eating usually occurs in solitude and may stop if interrupted by someone. When the binge is over, patients may go to sleep or vomit, either spontaneously or by insertion of a finger of spoon in the back of the throat.

While eating, the binges are pleasurable, but the patient experiences post-binge anguish and depressed mood.

When not combined with anorexia, the weight varies; patients usually do not lose and gain excessively, and the weight losses are never so extreme as to be life-threatening or incapacitating. However, bulimia occurs more often as a complication of anorexia nervosa.

Anorexia nervosa and bulimia are two separate conditions; however, they may coexist in the same person, usually in an older adolescent or young adult. Anorexia nervosa consists of a preoccupation with being thin; individuals suffering from it become thin to the point of emaciation. Bulimia consists of uncontrollable binge eating, usually of soft starchy foods that require little chewing. After the binge, patients often vomit or fall asleep. These patients are usually near normal weight.

When the two disorders occur together, the bulimia exists as a complication of the anorexia and the patient appears as a typical anorexic, thin to the point of emaciation.

SLEEPING IN SCHOOL

Nature of the Condition

There are three reasons why children fall asleep in school:

1. In a home in which children are permitted to stay awake much too late, having to wake up around 6:00 or 7:00 A.M. to get to school on time leaves them lacking sufficient sleep to satisfy the developmental needs for their age. They get sleepy during the day, usually right after lunch but sometimes even before noon. The amount of drowsiness varies from not paying attention to nodding, putting their heads down on their desks, and falling sound asleep.

2. Some children fall asleep as a reaction to stress. This bizarre emotional reaction has been reported in adults on the battlefields during actual combat. (A child's most frequent reaction to stress is stomachache or headache.) Stress-induced sleep is seen in children who are unhappy in school because of poor academic achievement or poor social adjustment.

3. *Narcolepsy* is an organic disorder somewhat related to epilepsy. True narcolepsy is very rare.

Diagnosis

Insufficient Sleep

1. Home visits to interview family members, sometimes not during school hours, are often necessary. One may find that the child stays awake till 11:00 P.M. or 12:00 midnight, occasionally till 1:00 or 2:00 A.M.

2. The child usually falls asleep at about the same time each day.

3. Mental and emotional health is usually normal in other aspects.

4. Most children in this category will be below the third grade.

Emotional Reaction

1. Home visits and other history will reveal sufficient sleep at home.

2. The child will fall asleep at a time when he or she is under stress. It may be in the classroom during arithmetic (if that is his or her worst subject) or on the playground if he or she has no friends.

3. It may occur at any age but most often in grades three to five.

4. It may occur after school or on weekends.

Narcolepsy

1. The child will fall asleep quite suddenly while doing something interesting.

2. It may occur while sitting or standing, but rarely will falling to the ground with injury occur as in a true epileptic attack.

3. Each attack lasts about the same length of time.

4. After awakening, the child is drowsy only for a short time.

5. Medical exam often shows an abnormal brain wave pattern.

6. Academic achievement and social adaptation is normal unless there are additional cognitive and/or emotional problems.

7. *Cataplexy,* a sudden loss of muscle tone, *sleep paralysis,* an inability to move while falling asleep, and *hypnagogic hallucinations,* frightening vivid dreams on awakening occur on rare occasions.

Treatment

The underlying cause will naturally suggest the proper treatment and management.

Medical treatment is limited to medication and, as this will be helpful in only a small percentage of cases, is rarely used.

Educational management consists of special classes, lessening educational demands, and occasionally tutoring. If the home situation is completely chaotic and nothing can be done to change it, some principals provide a quiet area where a kindergartener or first grader can take a one- or two-hour nap after lunch.

Emotional support can be provided by the school nurse, counselor, or teacher. This is always an important addition to any other method of management and often yields good results.

Role of the School Nurse

1. Home visits (this is one of the most important diagnostic steps; information gathered will be most helpful)
2. Consultation with parents
3. Referral to physician
4. Liaison between parents, physician, and school personnel
5. Monitoring and/or administering medication in those rare cases when it is prescribed for narcolepsy or emotional problems

PSYCHOACTIVE MEDICATIONS COMMONLY USED FOR CHILDREN

Amphetamines
- Desirable Effects
- Undesirable Effects

Phenothiazines
- Desirable Effects
- Undesirable Effects

Antidepressants
- Desirable Effects
- Undesirable Effects

Benzodiazepines
- Desirable Effects
- Undesirable Effects

Role of the School Nurse

Giving Medications in School
- Legal Implications
- Frequent Problems Concerning Medications
- Students Carrying and Giving Themselves Medicines

All of the drugs described in this chapter require a physican's prescription. They all have multiple adverse side effects. School staff in charge of monitoring them should have ready access to the *Physician's Desk Reference,* published by Medical Economics in Oradell, New Jersey.

The drugs described are only the ones most commonly used. Many more are available and occasionally used by some physicians.

In this chapter, the words *drugs* and *medications* are used synonymously. A psychoactive drug is one that is designed to have a primary effect on brain functioning. Many of them are prescribed for children in school and are designed to have their effects during school hours. Two examples are Mellaril and Ritalin. They are used to treat children with severe behavior disorders that require medication for their control.

Non-psychoactive drugs may have psychoactive side effects. For example, Dramamine, used for seasickness, on occasion makes a person sleepy though it is not classified as a psychoactive drug.

AMPHETAMINES

Ritalin	(generic name: methylphenidate)
Cylert	(generic name: pemoline)
Dexedrine	(generic name: dextro amphetamine)

Amphetamines are prescribed legitimately for only three conditions:

1. Hyperactivity (attentional deficit disorder)
2. Narcolepsy
3. Obesity (While some doctors still prescribe these drugs for obesity, such use is generally considered inappropriate.)

Desirable Effects

1. Decreased motor activity, impulsivity, and distractibility.
2. Increased attention span.

Undesirable Effects

1. Loss of appetite and poor weight gain. Unless severe, nothing needs to be done; the child will regain weight during summer vacation when medication is not given.
2. Nausea, stomachache, or headache.
3. Increased motor activity.
4. Frequent crying spells with little provocation.
5. Drowsiness.

Treatment of the above side effects consists of giving the medication after a meal, reducing the dose, or changing to a different form of amphetamine. If none of this relieves the undesirable symptoms, the medication may need to be stopped altogether.

6. Zombie-like state. This is rare. Treatment always consists of reducing the dose or changing the medication.
7. Tics. Whether or not tics can be caused or aggravated by amphetamines is controversial. As long as the possibility exists, the school nurse must be watchful and report any new tics or worsening of old ones to the parent and/or doctor.
8. Addiction. This never occurs as long as the drug is given in small, controlled doses.

Some of the amphetamines are long-acting; one dose given in the morning lasts all day. These are Dexedrine spansules, Cylert, and Ritalin-SR (sustained release). My preference is to start treatment with the short-acting drug to establish a baseline dose and to determine individual tolerance. The short-acting amphetamines usually require a morning dose between 7:00 and 8:00 A.M. and another dose between 11:00 A.M. and 12:00 noon. By the time the child gets home from school, the effects are over. Occasionally a child is so hyperactive that a third dose at about 3:00 or 4:00 P.M. will be necessary.

PHENOTHIAZINES

Thorazine   (generic name: chlorpromazine)
Stelazine   (generic name: trifluoperazine)
Mellaril   (generic name: thioridazine)

These drugs are often called the major tranquilizers in contrast to minor tranquilizers such as Valium and Librium. They are major because they produce more profound effects and are usually used for more serious conditions.

Their most common use in school children is for those whose behavior disorders are manifested by hostility, physical aggression, and violence.

Mellaril is occasionally used for hyperactivity if amphetamines do not help or cause serious undesirable side effects.

Desirable Effects

1. Decreased aggression and violence.
2. Decreased motor activity.

Undesirable Effects

1. Drowsiness and dryness of the mouth. These are expected effects and usually disappear in two or three weeks. If they persist or become severe, the dose may have to be reduced or the drug changed.
2. Weight gain, sluggish mood, and slow, foggy thinking.

These effects are usually dose-related; the larger the dose, the more likely they are to occur. Unfortunately, the dose required to control unacceptable behavior may in some cases cause all of the above-described undesirable side effects.

3. Further undesirable reactions. There are more than two pages of fine print in the PDR describing possible adverse side effects; some are very serious and occasionally permanent. Therefore, use of these medications requires careful consideration. Any child receiving them must be monitored closely.

Fortunately, in the low doses usually prescribed for behavior problems in children attending school, serious reactions are rare. Serious adverse side effects are more often seen in emotionally disturbed hospitalized patients who receive much higher doses.

ANTIDEPRESSANTS

Tofranil   (generic name: imipramine)
Norpramin   (generic name: desipramine)
Elavil   (generic name: amitryptyline)

These drugs are used primarily to treat depression in adults; their use in children is much less common. Tofranil is also used to treat bed wetting in children, but in the small doses used it is not supposed to have any psychoactive effects.

Desirable Effects

1. Elevation of mood.

Undesirable Effects

1. Dryness of mouth.
2. Sluggish mood and loss of fine motor control.
3. Further side effects. The PDR lists about as many serious side effects of the tricyclic antidepressant drugs as it does for the major tranquilizers (phenothiazines); therefore, the same warnings and instructions apply.

BENZODIAZEPINES

Librium   (generic name: chlordiazepoxide)
Valium   (generic name: diazepam)

These are two well known examples of the many minor tranquilizers available. They are usually called antianxiety drugs and are used for relief of tension and as sleeping pills. They do not help children with hyperactivity or aggressive behavior disturbances.

Desirable Effects

1. Relief of tension
2. General calming of mood

Undesirable Effects

1. Excessive drowsiness

These drugs are widely used in adults, much less so in children. The occurrence of serious side effects is rare; however, psychological addiction can occur easily, and these drugs should be used only when absolutely necessary.

Drowsiness is treated by reducing the dose and, if necessary, raising it very gradually in subsequent weeks.

ROLE OF THE SCHOOL NURSE

The school nurse should chart each dose of medication given at school. If the nurse is not at the school every day, the person who is delegated to give the medication should be instructed in the proper way to chart. The nurse should alert school personnel to children holding pills in their mouths and later spitting them out.

When possible, arrange for all of the medication to be given at home. The phenothiazene drugs have a longer duration of action and are more amenable to this mode of administration. Also, the long-acting amphetamines may be useful.

Take care that a child who is receiving legally prescribed medication is not mistaken for a drug abuser. Adverse side effects may make a child appear drowsy or "stoned," or to behave strangely.

Insist that a copy of the PDR be available for the nurse and other school personnel. The nurse acts as liaison between parent, child, and physician so that undesirable side effects or lack of therapeutic effects are promptly reported.

Two other helpful books are:

- *American Medical Association Drug Evaluations*
  535 N. Dearborn Street
  Chicago, IL 60610
- *Drug Information for the Health Care Provider*
  USP Convention, Inc.
  Order Processing Department
  12601 Twinbrook Parkway
  Rockville, MD 20852
  (800) 227-8772

GIVING MEDICATIONS IN SCHOOL

Only school nurses fully realize how such a simple act as giving a student medication can be fraught with legal problems, administrative complications, and adverse side effects.

Most schools require students to leave their medicines with the school nurse or another designated person, and to go get the dose when it is necessary, usually once a day, occasionally twice. This rule is difficult to enforce strictly, because many reliable students have chronic illnesses such as diabetes or asthma that require frequent medicines.

Each school should use some type of form on which to record the date and time medicine is given and the initials of the person giving it. Figure 15–1 gives a sample form.

This form should be kept *at the site* where the medicine is actually given, ideally in the nurse's clinic. It should be attached to the wall and easily accessible to facilitate recording.

Legal Implications

School districts usually require written parental permission and a physician's signed orders before allowing medication to be dispensed at school. In lieu of the doctor's order, some states permit medication

DAILY LOG FOR MEDICATION

School	Week of					Week of					Week of					Week of				
	Mon	Tue	Wed	Thu	Fri	Mon	Tue	Wed	Thu	Fri	Mon	Tue	Wed	Thu	Fri	Mon	Tue	Wed	Thu	Fri
Student ———— Dosage ———— Med. ———— Times ————																				
Student ———— Dosage ———— Med. ———— Times ————																				
Student ———— Dosage ———— Med. ———— Times ————																				
Student ———— Dosage ———— Med. ———— Times ————																				
Student ———— Dosage ———— Med. ———— Times ————																				
Student ———— Dosage ———— Med. ———— Times ————																				
Student ———— Dosage ———— Med. ———— Times ————																				

The person dispensing the medication signs his or her name in the block under the corresponding day of the week.

Figure 15–1. Daily Log for Medication

to be given in school if the medicine is in the original prescription bottle, properly labeled.

Most state nursing practice acts allow nurses to give medicines in or out of school only on a doctor's orders. The requirement for school nurses is the same as for other nurses. Also, no exceptions exist for nonprescription medicines. A teacher can give a child an aspirin; if the school nurse does so, she may have acted against the direction of her state practice act.

Frequent Problems Concerning Medications

• Students often come to school with aspirin or Tylenol wrapped in a tissue and no note from home. If the student knows the rules and tells the nurse, what should the nurse do, for example, when the student's menstrual cramps start and the nurse cannot locate the parents to get oral permission by telephone?

• Some diseases begin suddenly as an acute attack and require rapid administration of the first dose of medicine; otherwise, the attack can be severe. Three examples are asthma, diabetic insulin reaction, and migraine headache. High school teachers often don't know which child has a long-term illness and may be reluctant to excuse the child from class. But waiting forty-five minutes to bell time may be too long. The wheezing or blinding headache can become severe in just a few minutes. This is one reason doctors want some children to carry and give themselves their own medicine.

• Medication, prescription or not, that the doctor or parent has asked to be given "as needed" results in the nurse or other school person giving the medicine on student request. This is reasonable for responsible children, but problems arise with those who are not.

Students Carrying and Giving Themselves Medicines

Most principals do not want students to carry their own medicines and be solely responsible for taking it themselves when they need it. They give the following reasons:

• Students often trade medicines.
• Unprescribed or illegal drugs are carried.

- Students are found lethargic or excited with unknown pills in their pocket or purse—how can anyone at school know what to do?
- Students comply poorly with medicine schedules, even when a school nurse is monitoring them.

Whether to allow students to carry their own medicine has always been a difficult decision because doctors, when they make such a request, consider a different set of factors than do principals. The doctor envisions a responsible child and parent and thinks of the medicine's effect on the child's illness. The principal has experienced serious problems resulting from students' carrying their own medicines and is thinking about legal issues, equal treatment of all students, and drug abuse.

The official statement of the American Academy of Pediatrics, up to 1984, was that students should not carry their own medication. In 1984, the statement was changed to recommend that students carry their own medicine if so requested by their doctor. In my opinion, both statements were too dogmatic; there should be leeway for individual cases. We know that some students do trade medicines, take other's medicines, and carry illegal medicines. On the other hand, some students with certain illnesses should carry their own medicines and can do so safely. A reasonable compromise would contain the following sentence: "If the parent and physician agree that the student can be trusted with self-medication, permission of the principal must be obtained."

SECTION 16

DISORDERS OF LEARNING

Hyperactivity or Attention Deficit Disorder
- Nature of the Condition
- Treatment
- Schedule of Medication and When to Stop

Dyslexia
- Nature of the Disorder
- Diagnosis

Aphasia–Dysphasia

Perceptual Disorders

Minimal Brain Dysfunction

Lead Poisoning
- Learning Disability from Very Low Lead Blood Levels
- Role of the School Nurse

Nonstandard Remediation
- Vitamins
- Minerals
- Diets
- Hypoglycemia
- Allergy

231

- Patterning
- Visual Training
- Alpha-Wave Conditioning
- Sensory Integrative Therapy
- Perceptual–Motor Exercises
- Forms to Aid in the Diagnosis of ADD

Role of the School Nurse

Despite all the descriptions and definitions of "learning disability" there is still disagreement. What was gospel in earlier years has been discarded or is highly suspect today. The same fate will ultimately befall the truisms of today. There are many different categories of specialists who deal with this problem, and they differ radically. Whenever controversy exists in any field—history, science, or education—one can be sure that nobody has the true answer, or more likely that there is no single correct answer. Entire sections of the library are filled with articles on learning disability. I am only going to summarize those aspects of the problems that I know from personal experience are medically related.

Doctors first encounter the learning disabled child when a parent brings the child in for help. Since few doctors have had training in this subject, and since the usual physical examination shows nothing, the parent will be told that the child is normal. This would not be as likely to happen if proper communication preceded the referral. (For referral procedures see Section 1.) It is obvious that something is wrong when a bright child with normal vision and hearing, from a normal home, can't succeed in school. The school nurse or teacher should not stop with this answer from a doctor. The parents should be urged to get further consultation from a physician specialist or child psychologist knowledgeable about these matters. There is rarely need to consult a child psychiatrist at this stage.

HYPERACTIVITY OR ATTENTION DEFICIT DISORDER

Nature of the Condition

The most common types of learning disabilities are those which are associated with hyperactivity. Because the most significant symptom is a deficit in attention, the official nomenclature has been changed to *attention deficit disorder,* or ADD. However, some textbooks still refer to hyperactivity.

The following classification code is used:

ADD-H means hyperactivity is present.

ADD alone means hyperactivity is not present.

233

ADD-R means *residual:* an older child or adult who no longer has a motor problem, but still has an abnormally short attention span.

In the new *DSM-III-R-1987,* this condition is listed as a single diagnostic entity, Attention-deficit Hyperactivity Disorder (ADHD). The validity of ADD *without* hyperactivity is now considered questionable.

The symptoms vary according to age. Children aged five through nine always "have their motor running"—they are constantly climbing and running. Preadolescents are restless and fidgety. Adolescents tend toward impulsive social behavior such as going joy-riding instead of doing homework.

The diagnostic criteria, as listed in *DSM-III-R*, should be present for at least six months, begin before age seven, and exist to a greater degree than normal. They are as follows:

1. often fidgets with hands or feet or squirms in seat (in adolescents, may be limited to subjective feelings of restlessness)
2. has difficulty remaining seated when required to do so
3. is easily distracted by extraneous stimuli
4. has difficulty awaiting turn in games or group situations
5. often blurts out answers to questions before they have been completed
6. has difficulty following through on instructions from others (not due to oppositional behavior or failure of comprehension), e.g., fails to finish chores
7. has difficulty sustaining attention in tasks or play activities
8. often shifts from one uncompleted activity to another
9. has difficulty playing quietly
10. often talks excessively
11. often interrupts or intrudes on others, e.g., butts into other children's games
12. often does not seem to listen to what is being said to him or her
13. often loses things necessary for tasks or activities at school or at home (e.g., toys, pencils, books, assignments)

14. often engages in physically dangerous activities without considering possible consequences (not for the purpose of thrill-seeking), e.g., runs into street without looking

Critieria for severity of Attention-deficit Hyperactivity Disorder:

Mild: Few, if any, symptoms in excess of those required to make the diagnosis and only minimal or no impairment in school or social functioning.

Moderate: Symptoms or functional impairment intermediate between "mild" and "severe."

Severe: Many symptoms in excess of those required to make the diagnosis and significant and pervasive impairment in functioning at home and school and with peers.

The secondary characteristics which may develop as a result of psychological complications are:

1. Poor self-esteem; childhood depression
2. Anxiety neuroses
3. Juvenile delinquency
4. Alcoholism in adults

ADD occurs most often in boys and has some very distinctive features, but it is rare that any one child will exhibit all of these symptoms. For example, some children with distinct ADD have a good memory and learning ability and grow up emotionally healthy.

Some experts think they can recognize a potential ADD child at one year of age, but the younger the child, the more speculative the diagnosis. It is rare that preschool children need medication. Also, children with emotional problems or hearing problems may appear to have an attentional problem. Their treatment, of course, is entirely different.

Some children with ADD are born with certain innate personality characteristics that interfere with their social adjustment and lead to further maladaptive behavior. Most long-term followup studies reveal that children usually get over their hyperactivity by the fifth or sixth grade, but their attentional deficits may remain, they sometimes are poor readers, and they often make poor social adjustments. However, if the child is lucky enough to have good parental, medical, and educational support, there is a good chance of making it through the educational system to become a normal, successful adult.

Treatment

The usual medical approach in the United States is treatment with amphetamines, and the one most often prescribed is Ritalin. There is much controversy about the use of this type of drug. It has its ardent proponents and those dead set against it. Researchers have been developing tests to try to predict which children will improve with amphetamines. However, the present state of the art is such that the most reliable approach is to use all or part of a multidisciplinary team of teacher, doctor, school nurse, and psychologist. A carefully monitoried clinical trial will prove the effectiveness of medication. When children are handled in this manner, the results are usually conclusive in a short time. It is most important to have a built-in monitoring system so dosage can be adjusted or medication stopped if undesirable side effects or treatment failures are evidenced. Amphetamines control hyperactivity very well in about 60 percent of the cases and moderately well in another 20 percent. The remaining 20 percent are either unimproved or get worse.

Dosage, of course, must be left up to the prescribing physician. Undesirable side effects are usually not seen until the total daily dose approaches or exceeds 60 milligrams of Ritalin or 30 milligrams of Dexedrine for a five- to seven-year-old child.

Because of the many articles published in the lay press about the horrible effects of medication, many classroom teachers have strong prejudices against the use of any drug for any child with behavior or learning problems. While these teachers are undoubtedly well intentioned, they are doing many children a disservice. True, the teacher knows the child well from daily observation and may well question the diagnosis and argue the case directly with the others involved, but one should never undermine the parents' confidence in these professionals through individual objections. The hyperactive child who responds well to a relatively small dose of amphetamine is being aided in a manner similar to that of a child with diabetes who receives insulin. While the medication does not cure this child, it certainly enables him or her to lead a more normal life.

Schedule of Medication and When to Stop

There is still disagreement in two areas:

- *Should the child be under medication all day, every day, or just during school hours on school days?* Most doctors prescribe amphetamines only on school days, not on holidays or weekends, and recommend two doses a day: the 7:00 to 8:00 A.M. dose lasts until noon, and the noon dose until school is out. Some children have such severe symptoms that the medicine is continued on weekends, holidays, and summer vacation, and at times a 3:00 to 4:00 P.M. dose is needed to last until bedtime.

- *Should medication be stopped at the youngest possible age, or should it be continued to or through young adult life?* Most children stop taking Ritalin between sixth and eighth grade. Some doctors recommend it be taken as long as there is any academic or social problem; others say that in early adolescence, children develop reasoning ability and some can appreciate the benefits of *not* having to take medication. Even though the attention deficit remains, school achievement can be successful with increased motivation and persistence. In other words, "you can do it, but you have to work harder."

These decisions are highly individual; there can be no blanket rule. I favor the approach that recommends medicine twice a day on school days only, stopping at whatever grade the child can do well without it (usually sixth to ninth). Like most pediatricians, I have seen children who require afternoon doses, weekend and holiday doses, and who need to continue their medication through high school.

Standard Ritalin Versus Sustained Release

For children with Attention Deficit Disorder with Hyperactivity (ADD-H), the standard, short-acting, 10 mg Ritalin, twice a day, works better for my patients than the sustained release, 20 mg, given once a day. My practice is to start new ADD-H treatment with standard methylphenidate (Ritalin), given morning and Noon, about three and one-half to four hours apart. If an individual child exhibits difficulty taking a noon dose at school because of psychosocial or scheduling problems, then the long acting can be considered. I have not had consistently good results with any of the long-acting forms (SR Ritalin,

SR Dexedrine, or Cylert). Occasionally they work well and should be continued.

Cost is also a factor. None of the long-acting drugs are available in generic form.

It is wise never to treat ADD with medication alone. Classroom management is just as important. When the decision has been made to treat a hyperactive child with medication, it is helpful for the teacher to consider certain behavior modification techniques and minor alterations in instructional methods. Following is a list of guidelines from *A Pediatric Approach to Learning Disorders* by M. L. Levine, M.D.:

1. Begin and end each day with praise for the child. Many children with attention deficits have significantly diminished self-image and feel as if there is no chance for success in school.

2. Break up work into small units. Avoid lengthy instructions and assignments whose persistence far exceeds the child's demonstrated working capacity.

3. Have a secret way of signaling a child who is inattentive to the task at hand. It is not helpful to call on a chronically inattentive child who is caught staring out the window. This may be humiliating and is likely to increase anxiety, which will further drain attention.

4. Whenever possible, such children should be in small classrooms, and the teacher should try to offer individual attention. There should be an awareness that such children may learn more on a one-to-one basis in ten minutes than they do during two hours in a large classroom.

5. A minimum of background noise and visual stimulation is helpful. A classroom with 200 different pictures on the wall, a fish tank, a gerbil cage, four terrariums, and a multicolored mobile may offer more sensory data than an inattentive child can filter.

6. Following a consistent schedule can help provide organization for such a child. Children with attention deficits generally do not adapt well to major shifts in program content or order.

7. The teacher needs to be sensitive to peer abuse. Such children sometimes have associated social ineptitudes (excess silliness, grimacing, body posturing, or "coming on too strong" when approaching a new situation or new group of friends) that cause rejection by their peers. The impact can be minimized by helping the vulnerable child to save face.

8. Motivation can be increased by involving the student in a personal way. Puzzles, finding mistakes in other people's work,

and games of concentration might be tried. The child should be helped to plan his or her work through a dialogue with the teacher or other problem-solving strategies.

9. Regular meetings with the child to discuss behavioral and academic progress are important. Offer concrete methods for feedback and monitoring (for example, graphs, scoring systems, diaries).

10. After an understanding is reached between teacher and child with regard to the attention deficit, discussion should center around whether or not the child was "tuned in" or in control of his or her attention rather than whether he or she was "bad" or "good." The concern here is that if a child is called bad often enough, this will constitute a self-fulfilling prophecy!

DYSLEXIA

Nature of the Disorder

Dyslexia was described in the closing years of the last century by a British ophthalmologist. The word derives from the Greek *dys* ("abnormal") and *lexia* ("words" or "reading"). It was thought to be a separate entity because the child (or adult) seemed perfectly normal and bright otherwise. Factors such as hyperactivity, mental retardation, emotional disturbance, poor home environment, and lack of educational opportunity could be ruled out by tests or actual observation. At that time, experts were pretty much in agreement about who did and who did not have dyslexia.

Today, confusion reigns because all categories of experts insist on their own definitions. No one can fully agree, and some say there is no such thing as dyslexia. The National Advisory Committee on Dyslexia concluded that in view of the wide divergence of interpretation, the use of the term served no useful purpose (cited by Lerner in 1976). Any population of reading-deficient children (or adults) rarely shows similar etiology or clinical manifestations, as one would expect it would if this were any single condition.

In the confusion that has existed, various experts have postulated that individuals with dyslexia actually see words backwards (*was/saw, dog/god*). However, articulate, intelligent dyslexic adults report that their difficulty does not lie in the actual perception or "seeing" of the word or letter but in what their brain does with it after they see it. They speak of difficulty in following a line of print, finishing the end of one line, dropping down one space and beginning the next, keeping their place with small print, and so on. It is becoming increasingly evident that dyslexia is one of the perceptual or intracerebral processing deficits; not a deficit in seeing but rather associating what is seen with the proper brain connections, resulting in the ability to read and write smoothly, easily, and rapidly.

Diagnosis

In my experience in reviewing cases, observing children, and talking to teachers, the following conclusions seem likely:

1. There is an entity that can be called dyslexia.
2. It is quite rare.
3. It is a different type of disorder from attentional deficit disorder (hyperactivity) and requires different management.
4. A child who has moderate to severe and fairly obvious emotional disturbances, hyperactivity, deranged psychosocial situations, and/or lack of educational opportunities should not be diagnosed as dyslexic.
5. Dyslexia can occur in combination with the above problems.
6. The diagnosis should be reserved for those for whom it was intended in the first place—children who are obviously of average or above average intellectual capacity and who, at the age of eight to ten years, after adequate educational opportunity, still can hardly read and are usually very poor spellers and writers. It is in this group of individuals—child and adult—that, with appropriate testing, one can diagnose true dyslexics.

Many children six to ten years of age are poor readers, sometimes to a severe degree, because they have emotional disturbances, hyperactivity, or poor psychosocial environments. Many parents of retarded or emotionally disturbed children prefer to use the more socially acceptable diagnosis of dyslexia for their children.

APHASIA–DYSPHASIA

Classical *aphasia* results from cerebral hemorrhage (stroke) that destroys certain parts of the left temporal lobe of the brain—the language area. This causes the patient to lose the ability to speak, even though all of the functions associated with speech remain intact. Breath control, tongue and mouth movements, swallowing, and all of the other things we always do automatically and unthinkingly each and every time we speak, remain normal. Because the hemorrhage rarely limits itself to a tiny, exact brain area (there are no walls or membranes to hold back the blood), there is almost always destruction of surrounding brain tissue also, so frequently there are associated symptoms as well, such as difficulty in comprehension of speech and impaired writing skills. Neurologists usually think of aphasia as the loss of previously acquired normal speech.

The term *developmental dysphasia* implies that the pathology in the language area of the brain was present at birth or acquired by some unknown means in the early months of life; *dysphasia* means a mild form of aphasia. To date there are no known tests to demonstrate whether or not these children have left temporal lobe pathology. It is logical to guess, however, that when techniques do become available, some form of brain abnormality will be found.

Dysphasic children have not developed normal speech, and their problems are quite different from those of an adult with classical aphasia. Remediation procedures, therefore, must consider this difference. Speech and language therapists are always involved in the management of these children.

Before diagnosing developmental dysphasia, it is important to rule out other primary disorders that may cause disordered speech, such as moderately profound hearing loss (past or present), cleft palate, or mental retardation.

PERCEPTUAL DISORDERS

Dictionaries define *perception* as "the act or faculty of apprehending by means of the senses or of the mind; cognition; understanding." The verb is "to perceive" and the adjective is "perceptual." They all mean the same thing. In educational circles, however, the phrase *perceptual disorder* is used differently. Neurologists would substitute the phrase *cerebral processing disorder*.

Neurophysiologists speak of sensory nerve activity by which messages enter the brain through one of the sense organs (eyes, ears, nose, tongue, and touch) and motor nerve activity by which messages exit from the brain to direct muscle contraction or relaxation, thereby causing body movement. When the brain receives the sensory message, it calls into play large areas involving memory, intuition, feeling, opposing messages, and many other factors. It then automatically correlates and computes this multitude of input in order to send out the proper instructions so that the body will respond in an appropriate fashion to the original input message. The cerebral activity between reception and response is known as intracerebral processing. It is a most crucial and important part of brain activity. When this particular function does not work right, an individual is said to have a cerebral processing disorder. A perceptual disorder and a cerebral processing disorder are exactly the same thing. The disorder is not in how one perceives but rather in how the circuit connections of the brain computer have failed to work properly and in the usual fashion.

Educators and educational psychologists speak of various types of perceptual disorders. A *visual–motor* perceptual disorder is usually taken to mean poor eye–hand coordination, which causes poor copying ability, handwriting, and drawing. *Perceptual–motor* disorders refer to children who have poor gross and/or fine motor control and poor body coordination. Gross motor movement means moving the body or limbs through space. Fine motor movement refers to using the hands and fingers. *Auditory–perceptual* and *visual–perceptual* disorders have also been described. For each labeled perceptual disorder, various tests have been devised to diagnose the disorder and various exercises constructed to treat it. Fifteen or twenty years ago these tests and remediation exercises were popular. They still have some faithful followers. However, research and clinical experience have cast doubts on the effectiveness of tests that purport to diagnose these disorders and the exercises that are supposed to remediate them. Children with perceptual disorders undoubtedly have impaired learning ability, but just exactly which cerebral process is impaired is not known. At present, some of the specific processes being studied are sequencing ability, spatial arrangement ability, memory (both long- and short-term), and attention span. Neurologists are not even sure what part or parts of the brain control these functions.

In light of what is known after years of observations, most educators, pediatricians, and neurologists feel that the best measures to remediate perceptual handicaps are not by perceptual exercises but by dealing directly with the educational deficiencies through various special educational techniques. Some students need to postpone studying those subjects that cause undue frustration or emotional problems.

MINIMAL BRAIN DYSFUNCTION

At the present time, the term *MBD*—for *minimal brain dysfunction*—is rarely used. There have been many recent advances in diagnosis and categorization of the various types of learning disorders, perceptual disorders, attentional deficits, and so on. Therefore, the term MBD has been largely discarded in favor of a specific diagnosis for each child, such as disorders of sequencing, memory, spatial or temporal arrangement and attention.

However, MBD is so firmly entrenched in professional literature that an understanding of what it means is essential. Until the late 1950s, the predominant opinion was that if a child had normal intelligence and didn't learn, he or she had psychological problems. Toward the end of the decade, a prominent pediatric textbook added a new section entitled "Behavior Problems Associated with Organic Brain Damage." Children with short attention span, distractibility, impulsiveness, various perceptual difficulties, and several other symptoms were included under this heading. This set the stage for the decade of the 1960s, when organic–biological factors were rated of equal importance with emotional–psychological factors as causes of learning disabilities.

In about 1962, lacking conclusive evidence of actual brain damage, the concept of brain "dysfunction" was introduced, and though the initials remained the same the majority of experts began to use the term *minimal brain dysfunction* to describe the constellation of symptoms formerly described as minimal brain damage. In 1968, the First Annual Report of the National Advisory Committee on Handicapped Children proposed the following definition (cited in Wiederhold, 1974):

Children with special learning disabilities exhibit a disorder in one or more of the basic psychological processes involved in understanding or using spoken or written language. These may be manifested in disorders of listening, thinking, talking, reading, writing, spelling, or arithmetic. They include conditions that have been referred to as perceptual handicaps, brain injury, minimal brain dysfunction, dyslexia, developmental aphasia, etc. They do not include learning problems which are due primarily to visual, hearing, or motor handicaps, to mental retardation, emotional disturbance, or to environmental disadvantage.

The term *minimal* is unfortunate. It is used to differentiate this condition from the major brain disturbances in which there is obvious, gross pathology, such as cerebral palsy or major mental retardation, and in which pathology can often be seen with the naked eye and always on microscopic examination of the brain. On the contrary, examination of the brains of children with MBD who have died from unrelated causes appear normal to gross and microscopic examination. This does not mean there is no pathology; it only means that neuroscientists have not yet discovered how or where to look. Current research continues to disclose interesting findings.

There is certainly nothing minimal in those individuals who are truly afflicted with handicaps that affect them severely throughout their lifetimes. Many children with severe dyslexia are not properly diagnosed until ages twelve or fourteen. By this time they often have serious emotional problems that arise from repeated school failures. Many hyperkinetic children have, in addition to their learning problems and inability to sit still, serious difficulties learning how to socialize and are further damaged by negative feedback. They have experienced peer and adult rejection beginning at about three years of age, and their emotional developmental pattern is often adversely affected to a severe degree.

It is also unfortunate that the term *minimal* seems to be associated in the minds of many legislators with *minor* or *unimportant*. When they apportion funds, it is this category that is usually short-changed. Therefore, these children, who are most amenable to good remediation, get the least. Many followup studies, beginning decades ago, have shown that it is this group of children which eventually accounts for most of the young jail population. Funds properly applied to help this type of childhood school failure could often produce a healthy, happy, educated, tax-paying adult.

LEAD POISONING

When lead is combined with certain other chemicals and ingested or inhaled it is readily absorbed into body cells and causes either acute or chronic lead poisoning.

Acute: If large amounts of lead are ingested over a short period of time such as one to three weeks, headache, blurred vision, disorientation, and other signs of brain dysfunction appear. This type of poisoning is rare today. However, if untreated, it may end in coma and death.

Chronic: Children who ingest small amounts of lead over a period of months or years develop headaches, stomach aches, peripheral nerve weaknesses, confusion, poor cognitive abilities, poor nutrition and other signs of chronic illness. This clinical picture was seen in years past, especially in older northeastern cities where old houses were painted with leaded paint. (Toddlers would chew on the window sill.) Most paint no longer contains lead, so it is not the prime source now. (Some art supplies contain lead, however.) Now it comes primarily from automobile exhaust fumes from leaded gasoline and lead plumbing pipes and soldering. Electric water coolers may have lead tanks and connections.

Learning Disability from Very Low Lead Blood Levels

Since children's brains are still growing, it takes less lead to cause brain damage in a child than in an adult. At this time, the Center for Disease Control's standard for "acceptable blood lead level" is 25 mcg%. Below 25 mcg%, observable ill effects are not produced. However, recent research[1] shows that newborn babies with a cord blood lead level of 10–25 mcg% (from the mother) scored low on mental and cognitive tests when they were two years old. Other studies have confirmed this on older children.[2]

---

[1] Bellinger, et al., *New England Journal of Medicine*, April 23, 1987.

[2] Faust D et al, *Pediatrics*, November 1987.

Role of the School Nurse

Children categorized as learning disabled rarely come to the attention of the school nurse. However, low level lead poisoning may be suspected in some children who are not achieving at expected rates. The nurse may have the opportunity to alert the parent or their doctor to this possibility. Also, if there are water coolers in the school, they should be checked for unacceptable levels of lead output.

NONSTANDARD REMEDIATION

The chronic handicaps that adversely affect learning and acceptable behavior require such prolonged medical as well as educational intervention that parents are particularly vulnerable to the appeal of any method that offers a quick cure. The history of medicine is replete with such nostrums; there are more in existence today than ever before. It takes a combination of scientifically oriented doctors; well-controlled, double-blind studies; and, if medication is involved, the use of placebos to prove the effectiveness of any form of therapy. Such safeguards are just as important in the educational as in the medical treatment of children with learning disorders and other developmental disabilities.

Most pediatric neurologists, as well as doctors who specialize in behavioral and learning problems of children, favor direct special education remediation methods. It is particularly important that educational demands are not so great as to add to the child's emotional problems. The child needs to experience success through obtainable goals, trained teachers, and small class size.

On the other hand, parents need to have a role that they feel will, by their dedication, ameliorate their child's disability. They do not want to be told that acceptance is a major part of their role; they will resist this by grasping at every available alternative, and they will see in any change evidence that vindicates their faith, even though these changes occur more from elapsed time and parental attention than from the latest treatment regimen. Therefore, it is important to reassure parents that there is something that can be done and that their participation is necessary. This something is not "curing" the learning disability, but rather using educating techniques that acknowledge the child's limitations and utilize and build on the potential present in every child. The parents need medical and educational experts to identify what their particular child has to work with and what techniques to apply to develop these functions to their utmost. Given specific activities, the parent can be helped to resist false hopes. Even so, the hope for a normal child will be latently waiting to spring alive.

Remedial methods that are suspect in their effectiveness are those that are based on various vitamins, diets, perceptual training methods, hypoglycemia, patterning, and optical training methods. These "cures" are akin to many highly questionable and spurious medical treatments that have come and gone in past years. They are based on theories rejected by experts who judge them ineffective, but their proponents become quite defensive when challenged. Many testimonials and anecdotal case studies are offered as evidence, but objective researchers using the same techniques have failed to duplicate these claims of effectiveness.

Vitamins

There are still those who advocate treatment of learning disabilities with large doses of vitamins. Recognized medical authorities agree that this "orthomolecular" or "megavitamin" therapy has no benefit. It does have the definite potential danger of most large-dose vitamin regimes. Vitamins A, D, and E have well-known toxic effects. Even vitamin C, which some have advocated in large doses for the common cold, can cause kidney stones.

Minerals

Copper and zinc are two of the various minerals that have been recommended as treatments for learning disability. As with vitamins, minerals provide no proven beneficial effect despite claims to the contrary. Also, toxic side effects are well documented.

Diets

The Feingold diet enjoyed a brief period of popularity as treatment for hyperactive children. Its theoretical basis is that many foods and food dyes contain salicylates that cause hyperactivity in certain susceptible children.

Some of the earlier studies by other authorities were tentatively confirmatory, but all later work has failed to bear out the early optimism. It can now be stated that the diet is generally not helpful. The most that can be said is that it may be helpful in a small subset of hyperactive children. Besides, it is extremely difficult to prepare. The entire family must eat it if the child is expected to stay with it, and the child who already has a problem with peer relations is segregated even further during parties and snack times.

Hypoglycemia

Low blood sugar has been cited as a cause of learning disability. Though this is also unsubstantiated, hypoglycemia has become a "wastebasket" type of diagnosis for many common complaints of a vague behavioral or neurologic nature.

All physicians of considerable experience have seen patients with true hypoglycemia. It is both rare and serious. It must be very carefully diagnosed, usually under hospital conditions, and just as carefully treated. It is not to be considered as a cause of learning disability.

Allergy

Certain allergists state that some learning disorders are caused by allergies of the brain to certain specific foods or other substances. They have advocated allergic testing and desensitization treatments. They describe what has been called the *tension–fatigue* syndrome as a type of learning disability.

Again, none of this has been confirmed and is regarded as highly suspect by most medical experts.

Patterning

The patterning method, originating thirty years ago as treatment for mental retardation, cerebral palsy, learning disability, and a host of other disorders, is also known as the Doman-Delacato method. It enjoyed wide popularity for many years but is now rarely used. Objective medical investigation has proved this treatment of no benefit, and it is even considered fraudulent by some. It is usually recommended that the child be given the treatment for years, and treatment is very expensive. The false hopes given to the family delay the acceptance of the child's true condition and the initiation of realistic remedial educational methods.

Visual Training

Unfortunately, war has been declared along professional lines regarding the benefits of visual training in children with normal eyes to remediate learning disabilities. Many optometrists are sincerely dedicated to such treatment, while ophthalmologists and neurologists regard it as useless.

In brief, the two sides of this controversy present the following arguments:

Optometry	Ophthalmology
1. Children with reading problems are helped by glasses and/or eye exercises	1. If a child can see well (no refractive error) without glasses, glasses will not benefit his or her reading ability. Good readers can be cross-eyed, even near blind. They read well even though their noses practically touch the book.
2. *Seeing* involves use of eyes. *Vision* includes what the eyes see *plus* how the brain interprets this. Glasses can improve vision.	2. There is no difference between *seeing* and *vision*. A child without refractive error should not wear glasses. The eyes cannot be contributing to the reading problem.
3. Eye exercises will help a child read since tracking and certain other eye movements are an integral part of reading.	3. Exercises are beneficial only in certain children with abnormal eye muscles, such as in cross-eye. They do not improve reading ability.

The American Academy of Pediatrics and the American Association of Ophthalmology issued a joint statement expressing five major positions:

1. "Learning disability and dyslexia . . . require a multidisciplinary approach from medicine, education, and psychology in diagnosis and treatment. Eye care should never be instituted in isolation when a patient has a reading problem.
2. ". . . There is no peripheral eye defect which produces dyslexia and associated learning disabilities.
3. "No known scientific evidence supports claims for improving the academic abilities of learning-disabled or dyslexic children with treatment based solely on:
   a. visual training (muscle exercise, ocular pursuit, glasses)
   b. neurologic organization (laterality training, balance board, perceptual training)
4. "Excluding correctable refractive errors such as myopia, hyperopia, and astigmatism, glasses have no value in the specific treatment of dyslexia or other learning problems.
5. "The teaching of learning-disabled and dyslexic children is a problem of educational science."

Most optometrists do a limited assessment, focusing on visual and visual motor areas of functioning but not on auditory and language areas. Thus, even if an optometric evaluation should indicate a certain type of visual disability, it will not necessarily rule out the possibility of the child having other areas of disability. A full special educational evaluation should cover all areas of possible disability. It should also integrate the therapy into the full learning process (like remedial reading or math) to assist the child's performance within the classroom.

Alpha-Wave Conditioning

At one time biofeedback techniques were used experimentally for the alleviation of learning disability. Children suspected of having poorly organized alpha waves on an electroencephalogram were taught through feedback to control their alpha waves, and this was supposed to cure or help their learning disability. This, too, has been discarded.

Sensory Integrative Therapy

Sensory integrative therapy was advocated by a California occupational therapist, A. J. Ayres, in 1965. It was assumed that maximum integration of sensory stimuli would improve classroom performance. Examples of such exercises were: involving the sense of balance by postural changes such as spinning or skating; tactile stimulation like working puzzles, feeling vibrating brushes, etc.

This therapy is still practiced by some occupational therapists, and in some OT schools it is still taught as a useful technique. Pediatric and neurologic specialists, for the most part, do not agree that this is a useful technique. I predict that it will gradually fall by the wayside.

Perceptual–Motor Exercises

It has been noted that children with learning disabilities are often clumsy. Various researchers have developed physical exercises that are designed to aid the child's perception of his or her body parts—self-image in the anatomical sense. Remedial procedures include walking on a narrow board, using a balance board, trampoline exercises, rhythm exercises, and so on. Kephart has developed a theory that postulates a number of states through which a child must progress to regain all lost ground. This approach is somewhat similar to the Doman-Delacato method, at least in theory, and its effectiveness is unproved. The children, however, love it. Its greatest value lies in getting the reading-disabled child out of the classroom and into an area of the school where he or she cannot only have fun but also succeed. The perceptual–motor exercises, if judiciously used, can be done in the school itself, thereby simultaneously combined with and related to a remedial reading program. The major benefit in a program of positive experience of this type is likely the result of enhancement of the child's self-concept, so it also helps if the child feels that the reason for doing the exercises is to help him or her learn to read. It is just as important for the remedial reading program to be carefully structured so the child succeeds at this task as well, no matter how simple it is.

Summary

Caught in the middle of all the controversies are the teachers and parents. How do they know whom to believe? It is hardly possible for them to study all the literature in the field, so they have no basis for an informed decision. At the present state of our knowledge about learning disability, the best course to follow is one of healthy skepticism about any single approach, especially if it seems simplistic or is widely disputed.

There is evidence that indicates that approaches to reading that rely solely on visual, auditory, or kinesthetic training, but do not include some actual reading experience, may lead to negative attitudes toward reading in general. Therefore, it is important to steer an even course between nonreading approaches and academic approaches.

The best lesson to be learned from the foregoing material is that more and more ingenious remediation methods will undoubtedly be developed in the future. Educators as well as school nurses and physicians will need to exercise vigilance in their judgment. They will do well to join in a dialogue that pools their areas of expertise.

ROLE OF THE SCHOOL NURSE

Some of the suggested activities go beyond the traditional role of most school nurses. However, the activities suggested here are all performed by currently practicing school nurses and have been found to be helpful to both physician and school:

1. Monitor and, if possible, administer prescribed medication.

2. Interpret the medical aspects of the learning and/or behavior problem to educational personnel.

3. Observe classroom behavior. Is there evidence of hyperactivity, aggressive hostility, excessive withdrawal, or other unusual behaviors? The two forms at the end of this chapter are excellent behavioral checklists. The school nurse can make them available to the teacher. The advantage of the Conners Behavioral Checklist is its brevity. It should be filled out by the classroom teacher and an impartial observer such as the school nurse. It can then be given to the parent to show to the physician or, with parental permission, sent directly to the physician.

4. Maintain telephone contact with the physician. Physicians usually get their feedback only from the parents. An informed school nurse can furnish accurate medical or nursing information from the school as well. This dual reporting will help the child's physician serve the patient more effectively.

5. Conduct parent conferences at school and at home. Children with learning disabilities are usually bright in most cognitive areas, and, if the consultation process is unduly prolonged, it doesn't take children very long to receive the message that the parents cannot accept them as they are. This merely reaffirms their already held belief that they are not worth much, and makes the remediation efforts more difficult. Therefore, parents must guard against continual consultations with too many experts.

6. When appropriate, assist in development of the individual educational plan.

FORMS TO AID IN THE DIAGNOSIS OF ADD

Conners' Behavioral Checklist

Patient's name _____

Teacher's observations

Information obtained _____ by _____

Month   Day   Year

Observation	Degree of activity			
	Not at all	Just a little	Pretty much	Very much
1. Restless or overactive				✓
2. Excitable, impulsive				✓
3. Disturbs other children				✓
4. Fails to finish things he starts, short attention span				✓
5. Constantly fidgeting			✓	
6. Inattentive, easily distracted				✓
7. Demands must be met immediately; easily frustrated			✓	
8. Cries often and easily	✓			
9. Mood changes quickly and drastically		✓		
10. Temper outbursts, explosive and unpredictable behavior				✓

$$0 \quad + \quad 1 \quad + \quad 4 \quad + \quad 18 = 23$$

Other observations of teacher (use reverse side if more space is required)
Used with permission of C. Keith Conners.

The Conners' Behavioral Checklist, shown on page 253, is used to measure hyperactivity. It is not exact. It is meant to be used as a guide, and is especially useful in following a child for changes due to a change in home or school situation, or to assess drug therapy effectiveness. Sometimes it is helpful for an impartial observer, other than the child's teacher, to fill out the form after a classroom visit.

Place a check in the appropriate column. Then score: Each check in column 1 gets 0; 2 gets 1 point; 3 gets 2 points; column 4 gets 3 points per check. Add the sum of each column:

Total score of 20 or over is abnormal; 15–19 is suspect; and under 14 is normal. (*Please note that in the example shown the total is 23.*)

ADD Comprehensive Teacher's Rating Scale (ACTeRS)*

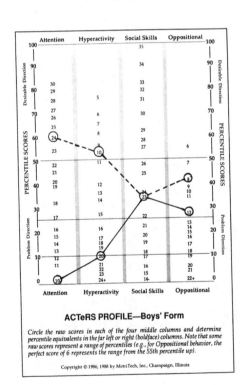

ACTeRS PROFILE—Boys' Form

Circle the raw scores in each of the four middle columns and determine percentile equivalents in the far left or right (boldface) columns. Note that some raw scores represent a range of percentiles (e.g., for Oppositional behavior, the perfect score of 6 represents the range from the 55th percentile up).

Copyright © 1986, 1988 by MetriTech, Inc., Champaign, Illinois

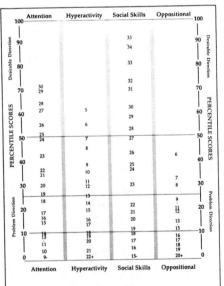

ACTeRS PROFILE—Girls' Form

Circle the raw scores in each of the four middle columns and determine percentile equivalents in the far left or right (boldface) columns. Note that some raw scores represent a range of percentiles (e.g., for Oppositional behavior, the perfect score of 6 represents the range from the 40th percentile up).

Copyright © 1986, 1988 by MetriTech, Inc., Champaign, Illinois

---

* This test is copyrighted by: Metritech Inc., 111 N. Market St., Champaign IL 61820. (217) 398-4868.

The ACTeRs PROFILE was developed by Dr. Rena Ullman and co-workers at the Institute for Child Behavior and Development at the University of Illinois at Urbana-Champaign.

It rates a child in four areas of behavior: (1) Attention; (2) hyperactivity; (3) social skills; and (4) oppositional behavior. Under each area of behavior, the teacher rates five or six items on a scale of 1 to 5. Examples of two items in each category are as follows:

Attention
  • Persists with tasks for reasonable amount of time
  • Follows a sequence of instructions

Hyperactivity
  • Extremely overactive (out of seat, "on the go")
  • Impulsive (acts or talks without thinking)

Social Skills
  • Behaves positively with peers/classmates
  • Skillful at making new friends

Oppositional behavior
  • Starts fights over nothing
  • Defies authority

After rating all the items and adding up the totals, the final score is placed on a graph. This is done before and after the child is placed on medication for ADD. The final graph appears as shown on page 254. In the sample shown, the solid line is before treatment and the dotted line after a good response to medication.

SECTION 17

HEALTH SCREENING PROGRAMS

257

Vision Screening
- Inspection
- Visual Acuity
- Excessive (Latent) Hyperopia
- Muscle Balance Testing for Ocular Alignment
- Treatment
- Depth Perception and Color Vision Testing

Hearing Screening
- School Procedures
- Measuring Decibel Levels
- Sweep check Screening
- Threshold Testing
- Referral Standards and Procedures

Dental Screening

School is the ideal place to conduct health screening, provided it is done without significant disruption of the students' educational schedules.

DEFINITION OF SCREENING

Screening evaluation must be differentiated from *diagnostic* evaluation. Screening is a relatively rapid evaluation of a large number of persons who are thought to be normal. A diagnostic exam is performed on a single person who is suspected of being abnormal: underweight, developmentally delayed, etc. An example of this confusion is the inappropriate use of the Denver Developmental Screening Test (DDST) as a diagnostic test in a child who is suspected, from observation, of being developmentally delayed.

The following terms are used in the statistical evaluation of screening tests:

1. *Validity.* The ability of the test to correctly identify the condition it is intended to detect.

2. *Sensitivity.* The ability of the test to correctly identify those persons who have the condition for which the screening is done. A test with high sensitivity will correctly identify 99 percent of positives. For example: If 100 persons with AIDS are screened with a test that is 99 percent sensitive, one out of 100 will show a negative test; fail to be identified).

3. *Specificity.* The ability of the test to correctly identify those persons who do not have the condition for which the screening is done. A test with high specificity will give a false negative reading only 1 percent of the time. For example: If 100 persons without AIDS are screened with a test that is 99 percent specific, one out of 100 will show a positive test (be incorrectly identified).

4. *Reliability.* The ability to reproduce the results on repeat testing or with other testers.

5. *Predictability.* The test's capacity to establish the proportion of the unscreened population who have the condition being screened for. For example: If a school screening program

identifies three out of 100 children correctly, and in the general population of that state the same ratio exists, the test is said to have good predictability.

CHOOSING WHICH PROGRAMS TO USE

Screening programs are costly and time consuming; therefore, they must be chosen carefully. No school district can perform all the health screening procedures available. Following are some guidelines to consider:

1. The condition being screened for should have a precise definition, agreed on by a large majority. Visual acuity of 20/20, for example, is universally accepted as normal. Dyslexia has no universally agreed-on definition. Therefore, vision screening tests are valuable. Dyslexia must be discovered through individual diagnostic exams.

2. The condition should be correctible or amenable to improvement.

3. The condition should not be a variation of normal.

4. Referral criteria should be clearly established.

5. Periodic evaluation and comparison with other schools and other testers should be maintained to minimize over- and under-referrals.

6. There should be adequate public and private referral sources to correct any defects uncovered. If not, efforts should first be directed at resource development. A major example is dental screening. Unless the children have access to dental care, screening and dental health education alone do not improve their mouths and teeth.

SCOLIOSIS SCREENING

Scoliosis means lateral or S-shaped curvature of the spine. It is now a mandatory school screening test in many states. With few exceptions, orthopedic surgeons and pediatricians feel it is a worthwhile screening test. The yield is low, but the children discovered to have scoliosis may be saved from extensive surgery or deformity later in life.

Technique

The screening procedure is described in detail in many textbooks and school and public health manuals. It is easy and quick, and, if carried out properly, accurate.

The child, dressed in shorts—plus bra or halter for girls—stands facing away from the seated examiner and bends over, palms together in a diving position, and touches the fingers to or near the toes. The examiner inspects the back from the neck to the lumbar region to see if one side protrudes. (See Figure 17–1.)

With experience, the examiner learns what degree of "hump" is abnormal. All children thought to require referral should be

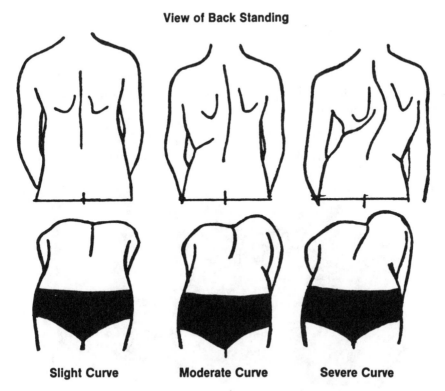

View of Back Standing

Slight Curve   Moderate Curve   Severe Curve

Figure 17–1. Scoliosis Screening.

rescreened after two to four weeks, preferably by another examiner, prior to referral to the doctor.

Screening should be done in the fifth or sixth grade, and again in the ninth or tenth grade.

A small handheld instrument is available that measures the degree of curve with a ball bearing. It is called a "Scoliometer" (see Figure 17–2) and is available from:

> Orthopedic Systems, Inc.
> 1897 National Avenue
> Hayward, CA 94545-1794
> (415) 785-1020
> TELEX 790471

Some screeners find the Scoliometer helpful, especially in measuring annual degrees of change of curvature in children whose scoliosis is minimal.

Screener Training

All nurses, athletic trainers, and teachers, who carry out scoliosis screening should go through a standardized training program. The program should have two parts:

1. Didactic presentation with movies and/or slides
2. Hands-on training supervised by an experienced screener

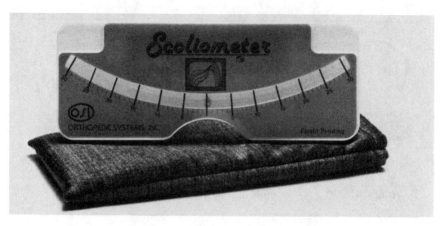

Figure 17–2. Scoliometer.

Orthopedic surgeons and experienced school nurses or trainers should take part in both aspects of the training.

Feedback is important. Every one or two years, all screeners should check their technique and referral criteria with either another screener or, preferably, an orthopedic surgeon. This is especially true where one or two screeners are working in isolation and receive little to no feedback from doctors to whom they refer.

Referral Rate

A 3 to 5 percent overall referral rate after the rescreen is considered acceptable. Consistent variations should be investigated. Not all children referred will require treatment; most only need to be followed by their doctor to see if the degree of curve gets bad enough to require bracing.

Single or Team Screeners

Some training programs instruct the screeners to look at the child's back while they are seated at the rear and again from the front (head). Two screeners can work more than twice as fast and, as an added benefit, confer on questionable cases. In some districts, a group of screeners go into a middle school of about 600 to 800 students and complete the screening in one to three hours. Principals prefer this method because the class disruption time is shorter.

One or more screeners can be trained for each campus, or an itinerant district team can be developed. An individual campus nurse can screen all the necessary children on her campus during a school year, a few at a time, with no class disruption. However, over-referral or missed cases are apt to result because the nurse works in isolation and gets little feedback to correct referral errors. My personal preference is for an itinerant team in a large district and individual nurse screeners for small districts.

Treatment

Most children referred require only skilled observation rather than definitive treatment because the scoliosis does not progress and get bad enough to require bracing.

The usual treatment is with a "Milwaukee Brace" worn 23 hours a day until the child's growth is completed. This is effective, but, as can be expected, compliance is poor. Recently, a brace has been developed which must be worn only during the night time hours. So far, the results are equal to the Milwaukee Brace and compliance is excellent.

There have been recent treatments with a relatively small battery-operated muscle stimulator taped to the skin of the back. Electrical stimulation causes the muscles on one side to constantly contract and thus gradually pull the spine into a straightened position. This gadget would be a boon to children if it could replace the brace. So far, it has worked in about half of the cases in which it has been tried.

Muscular training programs or specific "back" exercises neither prevent a curve from getting worse nor cure an existing one.

Controversy Over the Value of Screening

- Some scoliosis is nonprogressive. Referring these children may result in needless parental anxiety.
- The yield of children requiring actual bracing is low, and some say that screening is not cost effective.
- Each child referred needs full back X-rays, most of which don't show enough curve to require treatment. (Proper X-ray technique should shield the reproductive organs.)
- Children sent to chiropractors or other therapists may receive needless therapy.

Most school health authorities and orthopedists specializing in back problems recommend that school screening programs continue. I agree.

LABORATORY TESTS FOR MISCELLANEOUS CONDITIONS

There are several screening procedures now in use in school districts. All the tests described below are valuable as individual tests when done on children who have symptoms or history that lead one to suspect that the test may be abnormal. However, most of the recent controlled studies done to assess the value of these procedures have concluded that the yield is too low to consider them useful when they are done as screening tests on large groups of healthy children. The indications for the school nurse to perform any of them are as follows:

1. *Hemoglobin/hematocrit*—Weakness, pallor, or otherwise unexplained learning problems

2. *Urinalysis*—Frequency, burning, or wetting pants, especially if accompanied by other symptoms

3. *Throat culture*—Sore throat, fever, suspicious appearance on throat and/or on tonsils

4. *Blood lipid and sugar screening*—Positive family history of hypercholesterolemia or diabetes

When any of the tests are done in school, results must always be shared with parents and any abnormalities independently reported to the child's doctor.

TUBERCULIN SKIN TEST

The Centers for Disease Control, The American Thoracic Society, and The American College of Chest Physicians do not recommend screening skin tests of children of low-risk groups in communities of low prevalence of tuberculosis. They feel that a large number of children might be needlessly evaluated and treated for tuberculosis because of false positive reactions.

However, annual skin testing is recommended in children from groups in which one or more cases of tuberculosis have been reported. Such groups or families include native Americans and those who have come to this country from Asia, Africa, the Middle East, Latin America, or the Caribbean.

There are several multiple puncture skin tests available that are easy to use. The forearm should be grasped from below, the skin on the palm side of the forearm stretched slightly, the device pressed firmly into the skin, the forearm released, and then the device lifted away. This progression allows the skin to grasp the tines so a proper amount of tuberculin material is deposited into the skin. Puncture tests are all made to over-identify, so there is a high incidence of false positives; therefore, they should not be used in populations with a high prevalence of tuberculosis. All positives need to be retested with a standard intradermal Mantoux test.

The most reliable skin test is the intradermal Mantoux, using 0.1 ml of PPD. Whenever a multiple puncture test is used, all children testing positive should be retested using the Mantoux. To perform the Mantoux properly requires training and experience. If not done properly, the results are unreliable. Only the point of the needle, bevel side up, should be barely inserted under the skin so that the 0.1 ml, when injected, raises a clearly defined wheal about 5–8 mm in diameter.

HEIGHT-WEIGHT SCREENING

Height and weight screening is the simplest, quickest, and *one of the most important* screening programs available to a school nurse. Growth in height and weight is one of the most salient characteristics of normal children, and its absence should always be noted. Ideally, height and weight should be measured every year on all children. It is an ideal task to assign to a health aide or a student assistant. The procedure is simple and need not be described, but there are a few items that are helpful:

- The typical balance beam scale found in doctors' offices or health clubs is no more accurate than platform-with-dial spring scales. The important factor is gain or loss, so the child should be weighed on the same scale every time. If a child appears to have gained or lost one to three pounds as measured on a different scale, it is probably meaningless; neither scale is necessarily "correct." Scales of this type are not scientifically calibrated.

- Height measurement is best done with a yardstick attached to the wall and a triangle or square sliding down to rest on the top of the head, as shown in Figure 17–3. (CAUTION: Take shoes off and keep chin straight.) The sliding rod attached to a foldout flat metal strip that is found on a typical balance beam scale is not accurate. It may vary as much as an inch between readings.

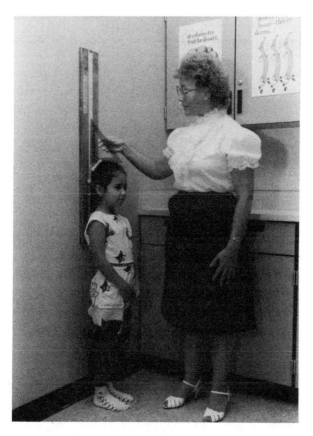

Figure 17–3. An accurate method of measuring height. (Note inaccuracy in picture: Heels should be against the wall.)

- Grids to plot height, weight, and head circumference on a graph are useful but time consuming. I recommend them only for students who appear, by inspection, to have a problem with height and weight. They are excellent as an educational aid for older children.

- All nurses *must* attach a table of normal heights and weights to the wall so they can refer to it constantly while weighing and measuring children.

- Children who are below the fifth percentile or above the ninety-fifth percentile or who fail to gain or grow over a year's time should be referred to their pediatrician.

BLOOD PRESSURE

Blood pressure measurement is part of a complete physical examination. School districts that are unable to provide total physical screening, with large numbers of students who rarely visit a doctor, may consider blood pressure screening. It is a low yield program, but for the few cases of hypertension (high blood pressure) discovered, early treatment is beneficial.

Hypertension prevalence rates vary with age, from 1 percent in young children to 15 percent in adolescence. With adolescents, most high readings return to normal after rest and remeasurement.

Here are some normal standards for blood pressure readings:

> 6 years and under 78/48–114/80
> 7–9 years 82/52–120/80
> 10–12 years 90/58–134/84
> 12–49 years 90/60–140/90
> 50 years and 90/60–160/95
> older

Figure 17–4 shows the percentiles of blood pressure measurements.

Warning

There are two important causes of false high blood pressure readings:

1. *Cuff size.* The cuff should be wide enough to cover two-thirds of the upper arm. "Cuff" refers to the *inner rubber bladder,* not the external cloth covering.

2. *Patient anxiety.* All elevated pressure readings should be repeated after the child rests for fifteen to twenty minutes. If it is still elevated, the test should be repeated in three to seven days.

Referral Standards

Readings over the ninety-fifth percentile for a given age, which persist on rescreening, should be referred. There are no hard and fast rules to follow. Here are some guidelines:

- Refer only those children whose pressure readings persist on two or three trials.

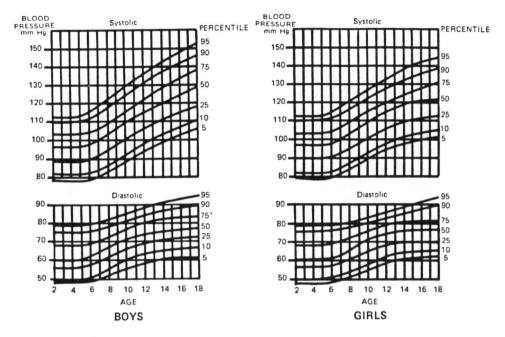

Figure 17–4. Percentiles of Blood Pressure Measurement.

- Refer children with diastolic pressures over 90.
- Refer children who have readings over the ninety-fifth percentile for age.
- Do not refer children with low blood pressure unless they have symptoms (fainting, dizziness, headache, etc.).

PHYSICAL EXAMINATION

The physical exam is normally done on individual children, not as a screening procedure on large groups of healthy children. In school, however, notably in the athletic program, it is often done as a screening procedure. In addition, some school nurses or nurse practitioners do screening physical exams, usually in the lower grades. In some states, the exams are mandatory at various grade levels. In my school district, screening exams are done at kindergarten or first grade, plus new entrants to grammar school.

From my experience, items to be remembered are as follows:

- Boys and girls should be done in separate groups.
- Failure to remove all clothing, except undershorts, is a common cause of missed abnormalities.
- Socks should be removed and the child asked to walk away and toward the examiner.
- Simple inspection of boys' genitalia is sufficient. With the child standing, the shorts can be lowered sufficiently to palpate the testicles and inspect the urinary meatus and foreskin. The foreskin should not be retracted. The inguinal ring need not be probed for with the examiner's finger.
- A pilonidal sinus or deep dimple should be looked for with the child standing and the cheeks of the buttocks slightly spread at the top.
- The most common previously overlooked, serious abnormality is undescended testicles.
- Items discovered during the exam that should not be referred because they rarely require any treatment are functional heart murmer, small varicocele or hydrocele, mild toeing in or out, and mild flat feet.

For many minor problems, the parent should be informed with a referral slip suggesting that the doctor look at it during the next regular visit; this saves the parent the cost of an office visit. Examples of minor problems are ear wax and minor gait problems.

VISION SCREENING

Without doubt, school health personnel spend more time performing vision and hearing screening than any other single activity. A complete vision screening program consists of six parts:

1. visual inspection of the eyes
2. visual acuity
3. testing for ocular alignment, such as cross eye or wall eye
4. excessive or latent hyperopis
5. depth perception
6. color vision

Inspection

This is an important part of the vision screen. Squint, sensitivity to light, redness of the eye, discolorations, abnormalities of the white or colored part of the eye (for example, coloboma, a defect of the iris), eczema of the eyelids, mild strabismus, and many other significant problems are often discovered. It can be done quickly without the child's being aware. Each vision screener should follow a brief checklist; after examining a few students, the procedure will become automatic. The reason that eye specialists prefer doing the visual acuity exam with the 10- or 20-foot Snellen chart is that it gives the screener the opportunity for this inspection. If the Titmus, telebinocular, or other similar machine is used, the examiner is not able to see the child's eyes.

Visual Acuity

The procedure for this part of the vision screen is well described in many state manuals and school procedure books. Therefore, only a few relevant factors will be emphasized here:

1. For reasons stated above, the 10- or 20-foot Snellen chart is recommended. For children who are difficult to test, I recommend the "Insta-Line" system made by the Good-Lite Co., 1540 Hannah Avenue, Forest Park, IL 60130. It allows the nurse to sit near and watch the child's face while she lights up a single letter or line on the lighted box containing the Snellen chart. It is expensive; each box costs about $500 to $600. (See Figure 17–5.)

2. For pre-kindergarten children, I recommend the STYCAR (HOTV symbols) or the "pre-literate" or "tumbling" *E*. STYCAR is an acronym for Screening Test for Young Children and Retardates.

3. The Titmus Vision Tester is widely used and gives an accurate enough reading of visual acuity. It can be used for testing convergence ability (which is required for binocular vision), depth perception, and excessive hyperopia. It is usually used by nurses whose clinic is too small or cluttered to use the Snellen. While children are using it, their eyes cannot be seen.

4. The Keystone Telebinocular was in vogue in the past but is not used much now. It is designed to perform many of the functions of the Titmus but is more complicated and not as useful in a school vision screening program.

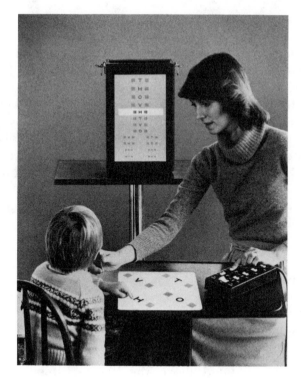

Figure 17–5. The "Insta-Line" system.

5. There are standards in each state for referring children to a vision specialist. The American Academy of Pediatrics School Health Guide recommends the following:
   a. Up to the fifth birthdate children should read a majority of the 20/40 line with each eye.
   b. after the fifth birthdate children should read a majority of the 20/30 line with each eye.
   c. a two-line difference between eyes, even in the normal range, should be referred.

6. Peeking and quickly memorizing the chart is rampant among school children. All vision testers should keep this in mind, especially in young children the first time they are screened, because many defects, if discovered early enough, can be cured. If missed on the first screen, the child may develop amblyopia and be permanently blind in one eye by the next screening exam.

7. Referral is made to vision specialists: ophthalmologists, who are MDs; and optometrists, who are not MDs, but are sufficiently

trained and well prepared to prescribe glasses. My preference is to refer to a vision specialist who neither dispenses (sells) glasses, nor is adjacent to or has a business interest in a store that does.

Excessive (Latent) Hyperopia

Small degrees of hyperopia are common in children; 75 percent of newborns are mildly so, and 50 percent still are at age sixteen. These children see and read perfectly well without glasses. If the hyperopia is severe, the accommodative power of the lens of the eye is insufficient, vision will be blurred, and the child will fail the vision screening test.

However, there is a small group of hyperopic children on the borderline who will pass the vision screening test; they can see well but must accommodate so much that their eyes tire, and they sometimes complain about their eyes or prefer not to read. To test these children, the school nurse can use a pair of 2.5 diopter plus lenses. A normal child will not be able to pass a standard Snellen test wearing these glasses; the chart will be too blurred. A child with moderate to severe hyperopia will pass the test easily, because this is the type lens used to correct hyperopia.

Some nurses perform this test on all children as part of the vision screening program. It is a low yield program, but some feel it is worthwhile because it takes so little time. I suggest it be done only in the elementary grades (K–3).

Muscle Balance Testing for Ocular Alignment

Deviation of the eye can be toward the nose (cross eye or eso-tropia) or away from the nose (wall eye or exotropia). Less commonly, the deviation is straight up or obliquely up. All forms are caused by excess pull of one of the eye muscles. The deviation is often seen when the child gazes into the distance without focusing on a single point.

When it is always the same eye that deviates, it is called *strabismus;* when the deviation alternates from one eye to the other, it is called *alternating strabismus.* Strabismus that begins at an early age, if uncorrected, leads to amblyopia; alternating strabismus does not.

There are several easy tests to detect mild strabismus. Two of the more common are the cover test and the pupillary reflex test. In the cover test, each eye is alternately covered while the student concentrates at a point 10 to 20 feet away with the uncovered eye. If the covered eye deviates, it will quickly move back to center when the cover is moved to the other eye. For the pupillary light reflex test, a child is asked to look at a light held 2 to 3 feet in front of his face. The light will be reflected as a pinpoint of light in the center of the pupil of each eye. If an eye is deviant, the pinpoint of light in that eye will be significantly off center.

Both these tests require some inservice training and practice to perform properly. They are a bit more difficult than it appears from reading about them. The inservice should be given by a consulting vision specialist or a nurse who is already proficient.

If either of the tests is abnormal, the child should be referred to a vision specialist. However, the nurse should be careful not to over-refer for minor deviations. *If the visual acuity is normal and equal* in both eyes, referral is not necessary.

Treatment

The time-honored treatment of strabismus is by surgery (lengthening or shortening one of the eye muscles). Unfortunately, not all surgery is successful; it depends on the type of strabismus. Oblique deviations are particularly difficult to correct.

Alternating strabismus usually requires no treatment. Also, if vision is not suppressed and the child is over seven or eight years old, surgery usually only helps improve the child's appearance.

Nonsurgical methods include patching the good eye, using special prismatic lenses, and many others. This is called orthoptic therapy. Treatment by an orthoptic technician should be supervised by a competent ophthalmologist, primarily to ensure that treatment is helping and that continued therapy is necessary.

Depth Perception and Color Vision Testing

Pediatricians, neurologists, and ophthalmologists agree that neither poor depth perception nor poor color vision adversely effect educational performance. Some educators disagree with this opinion. In any case, neither of these tests is done in most school screening programs.

Since the child with either of these two conditions may have limited job opportunities, my suggestion is that they both be performed as a class project during middle school health classes. The health teacher and the school nurse, with a doctor as a consultant, can make arrangements so that it is an educational experience for the student.

HEARING SCREENING

Hearing and vision screening are the two most popular school health programs. There are many methods of screening hearing in school children, but pure tone audiometry done by school nurses is the overwhelming favorite. State health departments often give courses for school nurses in screening audiometry.

Most state legislatures mandate hearing testing of school children, usually more frequently in the early years and every 2 to 4 years in later grades. Also, new enrollees are tested.

Background noise, also called *ambient* noise, is a problem at school; rarely do school nurses have soundproof (anechoic) rooms. Window air conditioners and large fans are the worst culprits and often force screening to begin at 25–30 dB (decibels) instead of the recommended 20 dB. This is bad practice and should be avoided. Large ear muffs to exclude ambient noise are not effective and are not recommended.

School Procedures

1. For children in first grade and below, preparatory classroom demonstrations of the entire procedure are valuable. The audiometer should be turned up loud enough to be heard by all the children when the tester holds up the earphones. The children should respond by holding up a finger when they hear the sound.

2. The tester should check the audiometer every day before use by testing herself or another adult with normal hearing. Audiometers should be calibrated every year, or more frequently if dropped.

3. Children should be brought to the testing area in small groups so there will be less confusion and ambient noise.

4. Glasses and large earrings should be removed, chewing gum disposed of, hair tucked out of the way, and the earphones fitted snugly over the ears.

Measuring Decibel Levels

Intensity (loudness) of sound is expressed in decibels (dB). Zero dB is the level of sound that can barely be heard by a normal young adult; it is not the absence of sound. This is why some children hear pure tones at −10 or −20 dB.

A tone's highness or lowness of pitch is expressed in Herz (Hz, also called frequency or cycles). Low-pitched tones tested are 125, 250, and 500 Hz; high tones are 4,000, 6,000 and, occasionally, 8,000 Hz.

Sweep Check Screening

Most nurses begin testing at 20, 25, or 30 dB (20 is recommended, if possible), depending on the ambient noise. Most programs recommend screening at 1,000, 2,000, and 4,000 Hz; some recommend 5,000 Hz also, as the final step. Each ear is tested separately. Children who can hear 20–30 dB in both ears at all frequencies are passed. If the child fails, screening should be repeated in two or three weeks before referral to a physician, because minor respiratory infections may temporarily depress hearing.

Threshold Testing

This test establishes the lowest dB at which sound can be heard at each Hz level. In school, the usual levels tested are 500, 1,000, 2,000, 4,000, and 6,000 Hz. At each level, the nurse starts at 0 dB and gradually goes up until the child first hears the sound. Then the sound is decreased in steps of 10 dB until it is no longer heard. Then the sound is increased in increments of 5 dB until the child hears it again. This is the threshold for the frequency (Hz level) being tested.

Referral Standards and Procedures

The sweep check is done first. Those who pass are not screened again for one to three years unless hearing failure is suspected. Those who fail two sweep checks, given three to four weeks apart, are given the threshold test. Those who fail the second sweep check and the threshold are referred. Some audiologists think that school nurses should not perform threshold tests, but most school nurses feel they can do them well.

The levels at which a child fails the test are not rigidly defined, but all agree that children who cannot hear 30 dB at any single frequency (Hz) should be referred. Nobody recommends referral of a child who hears at 20 dB or better. The quieter the room, the lower the dB level that should be referred. Most state health departments issue exact referral standards.

There is some disagreement whether a child who can only hear at 20 dB or louder is at higher risk for learning problems. Most pediatricians feel that if a child can hear the spoken voice, learning will be normal, but some audiologists feel that children with a 25–30 dB hearing loss have more learning problems because they don't hear key words or sounds. Because there are so many other variable factors, this question is difficult to answer. For example, poor children have more hearing loss and also more learning difficulties. Is the learning problem associated with the hazards of poverty or is it due to hearing loss?

Children who need to be referred should be sent to a physician, preferably a pediatrician or ear specialist who is knowledgeable about children's hearing problems (not all are) and who is able to deal skillfully with children.

Most hearing loss in children is due to middle ear disease (otitis media) and is called a *conductive* loss. In adults the loss is usually due to repeated exposure to loud noises or degenerative inner ear disease and is called a *sensori-neural* loss. Often the hearing loss is due to some of both and is called a *mixed* hearing loss. Examples of audiograms are shown on the next page.

Impedance Bridge or Tympanometer

This instrument is useful, in a doctor's office, to assist in the diagnosis of chronic serous otitis media in individual children. It is used in conjunction with the appearance of the tympanic membrane, pneumatic otoscopy to see if the ear drum is mobile, and the results of the pure tone audiogram. With the use of all four modalities, a good treatment decision can be made.

Unfortunately, the impedance bridge, which is easy to use, has found its way into school hearing screening programs. When used as a single modality to screen large numbers of children, the result is over-referral, because the test has high sensitivity and low specificity. Because serous otitis is often treated by placing tympanostomy tubes in the ear drum, many doctors now think that impedance screening in

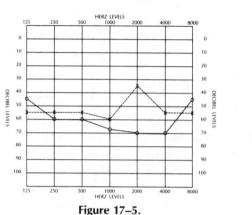

Figure 17–5.
Conductive Hearing Loss

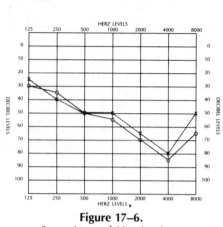

Figure 17–6.
Sensori-neural Hearing Loss

schools results in large numbers of needless tympanostomy tube placements. I have heard both sides of this matter for many years and have seen the impedance bridge used extensively in my school district. My conclusion is that it should not be used in hearing screening programs.

DENTAL SCREENING

Screening and education, by themselves, do not lead to a healthier mouth or longevity of the teeth. Dental prophylaxis (scaling, cleaning, and flossing), fluoride rinse, dental sealants, and repair of diseased teeth all contribute to healthy teeth. When community and private resources are available to provide these services, a dental screening program will be helpful in discovering the children who need to be sent to the dentist and dental hygienist. Until such services are available, all efforts should be directed toward providing them.

INJURIES

Inury to Internal Organs
- Stab: Penetrating Injury
- Blow: Blunt Injury

Eye Injuries

Head Injuries
- Nature of the condition
  —Scalp
  —Skull Fracture
  —Brain Damage
- Symptoms of Concussion
  —Severe
  —Mild
- Diagnosis
- Treatment
- School Relevance

Intracranial Hemorrhage
- Nature of the Condition
- Symptoms and Diagnosis
- Protocol

Lacerations of the Skin
- Nature of the Condition
- Treatment and School Relevance
  —Pain
  —Bleeding

—Prevention of Infection
—Dressing
—Sutures
—Booster Shots

Puncture Wounds of the Skin

Fractures
- Nature of the Condition
- Symptoms
- Treatment and Diagnosis

Dislocations
- Nature of the Condition
- Symptoms
- Treatment
- Role of the School Nurse

Arm and Leg Injuries: Sprain and Strain
- Nature of the Condition
- Symptoms
- Treatment

Bruise
- Nature of the Condition
- Symptoms
- Diagnosis
- Treatment
- Role of the School Nurse

Muscle and Joint Pains—Not Injury-Related
- Nature of the Condition
- Symptoms
- Diagnosis
- Treatment
- Role of the School Nurse

Burns
- Nature of the Condition and Classification Treatment

INJURY TO INTERNAL ORGANS

Stab: Penetrating Injury

Stab wounds of the chest or abdomen are extremely rare at most schools, the diagnosis is obvious, and there is never any doubt about what to do—immediate evacuation to the nearest hospital emergency room. If there is sufficient time, a large padded compression bandage may be applied, but not if it causes a delay in transfer to the hospital.

The parents should be notified after evacuation arrangements are made. If there is reason to suspect an ambulance will take more than a very few minutes, the school principal should take the initiative and have school personnel transport the child immediately.

Blow: Blunt Injury

Nature of the Condition

Injury to an internal organ from a nonpenetrating blow with a blunt object such as a rock, fist, or baseball bat is called a blunt injury. (See Figure 18-1.) There will be a bruise, large or small, on the chest or abdomen where the child was struck, but the seriousness lies in the damage to the internal organs—the abdominal organs, heart, or lungs.

Abdomen

A severe blow to the front of the abdomen can cause rupture or bleeding of the liver, spleen, stomach, or urinary bladder. A blow in the back may cause rupture of the kidneys. The initial blow will, of course, cause severe pain and often knock the wind out of the recipient of the blow. However, the initial symptoms may go away after a relatively short time, less than an hour in most cases. If there is no internal organ damage, no further symptoms will appear.

Rupture of an internal organ, however, can be very serious and may be missed if not suspected and watched for. The primary problem caused by a ruptured spleen or liver is bleeding into the abdominal

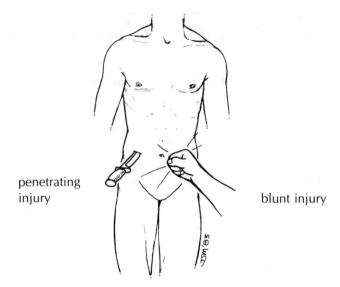

penetrating
injury

blunt injury

Figure 18–1. Penetrating and blunt injuries.

cavity in large enough amounts to cause the child to go into a state of shock and die unless an operation is performed to tie off the bleeding blood vessels. If the stomach or urinary bladder is ruptured, the problem is compounded by toxic material escaping into the abdominal cavity causing peritonitis. This is apt to cause marked abdominal pain sooner.

Chest

The lungs or the heart may be damaged following a severe blow to the chest. The period between injury and onset of symptoms is usually less than ten minutes. The cause of the symptoms is usually the same as in abdominal organ injury—bleeding. In the chest the excess blood compresses the lung and/or heart, thus impeding their function. If the blow is severe enough, the lung may actually be torn by a fractured rib, and then the escape of air from the torn lung adds to the difficulty. If this should happen, it would resemble a penetrating injury.

Symptoms of Blunt Injury to Abdominal Organ

1. History of blow to the abdomen.
2. Apparent recovery in relatively short time

3. Gradual onset, two to six hours later, of symptoms of shock: weakness, dizziness, sweating, rapid weak pulse and respiration, gradual loss of consciousness, dilated pupils of the eye, deepening unconsciousness leading to coma and death

Symptoms of Blunt Injury to Chest (Lung or Heart)

1. Rapid respiration
2. Apprehension and fright from not being able to catch breath
3. Blueness around the lips
4. Rapid pulse
5. Gradual loss of consciousness in severe cases

Treatment

1. Observe child in clinic for twenty to thirty minutes.
2. Place in position of comfort.
3. If no further symptoms appear, allow child to go to class.

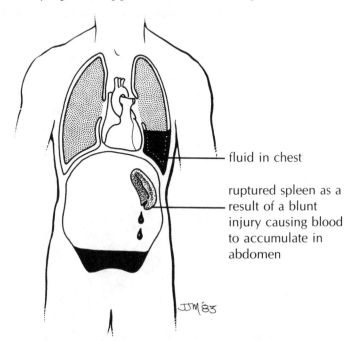

fluid in chest

ruptured spleen as a result of a blunt injury causing blood to accumulate in abdomen

Figure 18–2. Fluid or blood in chest and/or abdomen.

4. Check with teacher in one or two hours.

5. A ruptured stomach or bladder will usually result from a very severe blow, and the pain will be so severe that the child obviously needs immediate medical attention by a physician.

6. Injuries to internal organs result from blows of more than average severity. (See Figure 18–2.) Suspicious observation is necessary to alert one to the possibility. Delays in diagnosis are made when the child fails to report the accident or if the possibility is not considered at all.

EYE INJURIES

There are many ways for an eye to be injured: by a blow, a cut, a penetrating injury, or a burn. The child will hold the hand over the eye, usually crying and complaining of pain or rubbing the eye excessively. Tape a four by four inch gauze flat over the eye and send the child to the eye specialist immediately.

There are two types of eye injury that are serious but may escape detection by the school nurse or teacher unless suspected:

1. A blunt blow to the eyeball, such as with a baseball or smooth round rock, may cause an injury to the cornea and anterior chamber (front part of the eyeball). The pain subsides after a relatively short time, but the cornea may be damaged and a small amount of blood may collect in the anterior chamber. (See Figure 18–3.) If significant corneal injury is present, vision will be blurred. The only sure way to detect this is to test the child's visual acuity, preferably on the Snellen

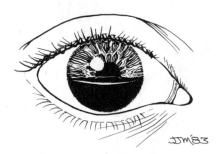

Figure 18–3. Blood (or other fluid) in anterior chamber.

Test Chart. If the test chart is not available, the child should read letters in a book with one eye at a time. Vision should be equal in both eyes. If vision in the injured eye is poor or blurred, the child should be referred to an eye specialist immediately.

2. A penetrating injury of the eyeball can be caused by a wire or nail. The only thing visible on the outside may be a tiny cut on the upper or lower lid, and a stoic child may not complain very much. If there is any suspicion that penetration could have occurred, refer to the doctor immediately.

HEAD INJURIES

Nature of the Condition

Head injuries are classified as bruises of the scalp, skull fractures, and damage to the brain itself.

Scalp

A bruise of the scalp is caused by a light blow that usually causes no skull fracture, brain damage, or loss of consciousness. A characteristic and mildly painful *hematoma* ("goose egg" or "pump knot") is seen. (See Figure 18–4.) Ice is the best treatment; pressure is not necessary. If there is no concussion or loss of consciousness, no further treatment is necessary. The swelling usually lasts several days.

Skull Fracture

Skull fractures are of two principal varieties: linear and depressed. *Linear fractures* look, on X-ray, like a cracked egg shell with both edges occupying about the same level as before the fracture. (See Figure 18–5.) They are caused by a relatively mild blow to the head. The blow causes pain, but the fracture itself heals with no special treatment. A *depressed skull fracture* does not mean the patient is depressed; it means a fragment of bone is pressing down on the brain such as might occur if someone were hit on the head with a hammer. This is very serious and requires urgent treatment. (See Figure 18–6.)

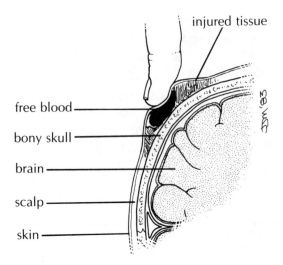

Figure 18–4. Hematoma of scalp. (The free blood under the skin feels soft and mushy. The injured tissue is swollen and hard, and a ridge can be felt (indicated by finger). This is often mistaken for a depressed skull fracture.)

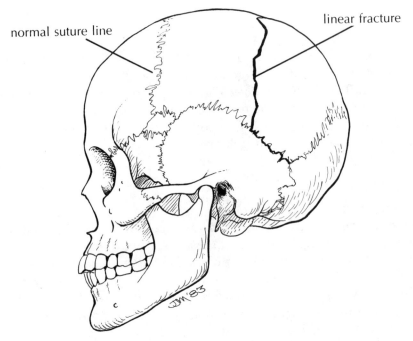

Figure 18–5. Linear skull fracture.

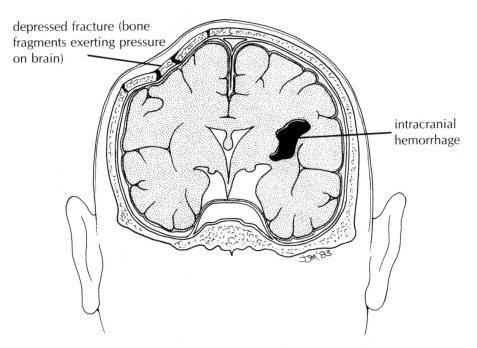

depressed fracture (bone fragments exerting pressure on brain)

intracranial hemorrhage

Figure 18–6. Depressed skull fracture with intracranial hemorrhage.

Brain Damage

Damage to the brain itself is classified as follows:

1. *Laceration.* This is an actual cut or crushing injury, always accompanied by skull fractures.

2. *Contusion.* A rupture of small blood vessels inside the brain occurs. The leakage of blood destroys the surrounding brain tissue and is usually accompanied by skull fracture.

Both contusion and laceration result from severe head injury, are accompanied by loss of consciousness, and are never treated at school. Both require immediate evacuation to the nearest hospital emergency room.

3. *Concussion.* Of the three types of brain injury, this is the least severe. When a football player or a boxer "sees stars" or "has his bell rung," he has suffered a concussion. A concussion can be very mild, requiring only a short rest period, or it can be quite severe, requiring a day or two of rest in bed. If one were able to look at the brain after a mild concussion, nothing would be seen. The symptoms are caused by the brain being "shaken up."

Symptoms of Concussion

Severe

Loss of consciousness is the most important of all symptoms and must be assessed most carefully. If the student is deeply unconscious and cannot be awakened, it indicates a severe concussion. The more dilated the pupils, the more severe the concussion. Unequal pupils also have a serious import. At first the pulse and respiration may be rapid, but with deepening unconsciousness they will become slower (Figure 18–7.) Vomiting always indicates a more severe concussion. There can be loss of memory for recent events on awakening (retrograde amnesia). Many children also suffer an antero grade amnesia—loss of memory of events occurring shortly after the concussion. This must be specifically inquired about or it will be missed.

Mild

A brief period of dizziness and/or disorientation occurs. There is a quick return to normality—the child may not remember what happened.

Diagnosis

A scalp bruise is diagnosed by inspection. Skull fracture can only be diagnosed by X-ray. Brain contusion and lacerations follow severe

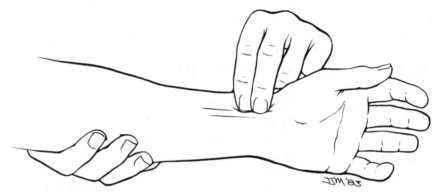

Figure 18–7. Taking the pulse.

head injury and will always be evacuated to a hospital for diagnosis. Concussion must always be strongly suspected following any blow to the head that causes momentary confusion, dizziness, or temporary unconsciousness.

Treatment

Concussion is the only important head injury that frequently requires school treatment. The cardinal principal of treatment is to prevent further injury to the head by an absolute prohibition of further physical activity for the rest of the day; in more severe concussion, as the doctor orders. It is well known that a second concussion soon after the first often leads to much more serious brain injury. The student should lie quietly for a few minutes with the head slightly elevated and, if it is a mild concussion, may then be allowed to sit. If the child remains asymptomatic, he or she may go back to class with a warning to the teacher to be alert.

Students with more severe concussion with a measurable period of unconsciousness should be evaluated by a physician.

Parents should always be notified in all types of concussion.

School Relevance

Normally, a mild concussion will cause no special problem; the child will rest and be perfectly normal later. There is, however, one notable exception—a football game. It is quite common for a high school player to suffer a mild concussion and continue to play, either because the student doesn't report it to the coach or trainer, or because, if reported, it is not regarded with sufficient seriousness and the student is allowed to play again during that same game.

Several organizations, such as the American Medical Association and the American Academy of Pediatrics, have formulated some fairly simple guidelines that all schools should follow:

One concussion—out of the game
Two concussions—out for the season
Three concussions—out for school career

This would prevent many deaths from head injuries, which occur every year in the United States during secondary school athletic contests.

INTRACRANIAL HEMORRHAGE

Nature of the Condition

On occasion, a blow to the head will cause rupture of a blood vessel between the brain and bony skull without causing any direct damage to the brain tissue or skull fracture. This is very serious, because blood can collect rapidly and cause deeper and deeper unconsciousness from continually increasing pressure on the brain. (See Figure 18–8.)

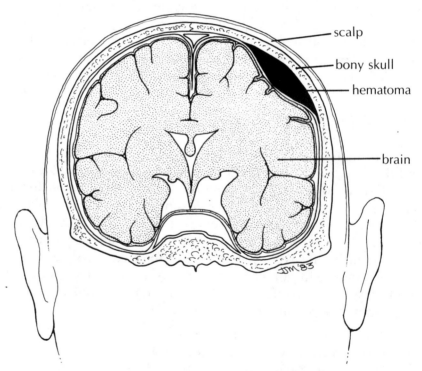

Figure 18–8. Subdural hematoma. (There is no skull fracture or brain damage. The blood collects as a result of a blow on the head, which causes rupture of small blood vessels.)

Symptoms and Diagnosis

All of the symptoms listed under concussion may be present.

There is one special type of intracranial hemorrhage, called subdural or epidural bleeding, which is characterized by a relatively brief period of unconsciousness followed by awakening and seeming normality. Several hours or days later, however, because of continued slow bleeding, the student may exhibit unusual behavior or slow lapse into unconsciousness again. This second period of unconsciousness has grave implications.

Protocol

The following sheet should be posted for all school personnel to see.

HEAD INJURY

Protocol:

1. Classify the injury as mild, moderate, or severe by the following criteria:
   a. State of consciousness (ranging from complete loss to fully alert)
   b. Vomiting
   c. Unequal size of the pupils of the eyes
   d. Unusually rapid or slow pulse rate
2. If any of the above four signs are distinctly abnormal, the child should be referred to a physician or emergency room immediately.
3. If the child is slightly woozy, but all other finds are normal, notify parents to take child to the doctor.
4. If all findings are normal, have the student rest in the clinic for 15–30 minutes, the length of time depending on the severity of the head injury and appearance of the child, and then allow child to return to class.
5. Ask the teacher to give you a report on the child's status in one hour.
6. Check child at the end of school day.
7. Notify parents by phone and in writing (see form below) of what happened and what to watch for. While the child was being observed at school, if the symptoms were to any degree more than the bare minimum, the school nurse should insist that parents get followup instructions from a physician.

**FORM TO BE GIVEN TO PARENTS WHEN
CHILD HAS HEAD INJURY**

Dear Parent:

Today _____ received an injury to the head. Your child was seen in the clinic and had no problems at that time, but you should watch for any of the following symptoms:

1. Severe headache
2. Nausea and/or vomiting
3. Double vision, blurred vision, or pupils of different sizes
4. Loss of muscle coordination, such as falling down, walking strangely, or staggering
5. Any unusual behavior such as being confused, breathing irregularly, or dizziness
6. Convulsion
7. Bleeding or discharge from an ear

If child was a little dizzy or foggy, vomited, or showed any of the other above signs, child should be checked carefully at bedtime and awakened at midnight (if bedtime is between 8:00 and 9:00 P.M.) to be sure he/she can be awakened and seems normal.

CONTACT YOUR DOCTOR OR EMERGENCY ROOM IF YOU NOTICE ANY OF THE ABOVE SYMPTOMS

_____   _____
School Nurse   School phone number

LACERATIONS OF THE SKIN

Nature of the Condition

Emergency treatment and later management of skin lacerations depend entirely on the nature of the wound, which may be clean and straight or dirty and jagged. Because of a greater blood supply, lacerations of the face and scalp usually bleed more profusely than those on other body parts. This greater blood supply, however, leads to better healing.

Treatment and School Relevance

Pain

Most lacerations seen at school are not very severe and rarely require medication to control pain. If the pain is severe, a physician must be consulted.

Bleeding

The best way to control bleeding is to place a gauze flat directly on the cut and press firmly with a finger or the palm of the hand. (See Figure 18–9.) After three to five minutes of pressure, the bleeding will usually stop.

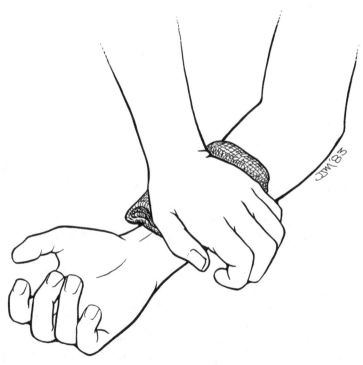

Figure 18–9. Applying pressure to large bleeding surface. (Amount of pressure should only be enough to stop bleeding—no more.)

Pressure over pressure points is often advocated in some books on first aid. This is rarely effective in slowing the blood flow.

Tourniquet application is controversial because, if applied too tightly and left on too long, the fingertips or toes may become gangrenous from lack of blood supply. On the other hand, for severe bleeding a tight tourniquet is absolutely essential. What is safe? For severe bleeding, especially arterial bleeding in which blood is spurting, apply a tight tourniquet 1 or 2 inches above the wound, note the time, and never leave it on for more than ten or fifteen minutes. The patient must be immediately evacuated to an emergency medical facility.

Prevention of Infection

If the wound becomes infected, the resulting scar will be larger. Copious amounts of soap and water should be applied to wash out all dirt and other contaminating materials. This may be a bit painful at first, but it is highly necessary. The water should be lukewarm and may be running from a tap or in a soaking basin. Germicidal or plain soap is beneficial

Merthiolate, mercurochrome, or other skin antiseptics cannot be relied on to prevent infection. Iodine is quite painful and it and other strong antiseptics impede the growth of fibroblasts, the new cells that grow out from the edges of the wound and heal it.

Dressing

Small cuts, after cleansing, only require an adhesive bandage. The bandage should be changed and the cut washed with soap and water daily until almost completely healed.

Larger cuts should be covered with a nonsticking gauze flat and adhesive tape and then referred to a physician right away, not at the end of the school day.

To make a butterfly tape dressing, adhesive tape can be cut to pull the two edges of the skin together so that, on healing, the scar is narrower and sutures are not necessary. There are two ways to do this. (See Figures 18–10 and 18–11.) This procedure is especially useful for jagged cuts that are incurred under contaminated, dirty conditions and are likely to get infected. By leaving the wound partly open, an abscess with trapped pus will not form underneath.

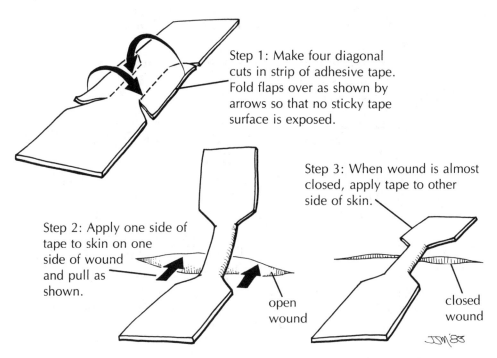

Step 1: Make four diagonal cuts in strip of adhesive tape. Fold flaps over as shown by arrows so that no sticky tape surface is exposed.

Step 3: When wound is almost closed, apply tape to other side of skin.

Step 2: Apply one side of tape to skin on one side of wound and pull as shown.

open wound

closed wound

Figure 18–10. Adhesive tape strip butterfly dressing. (Size is usually about 3/4 inch in width and 2 to 3 inches in length.)

Sutures

Whether or not a cut will require stitches is a highly individual matter. Several factors must be considered.

1. Size and shape
    a. Jagged, irregular cuts or cuts longer than 1 inch, with the

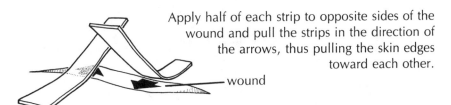

Apply half of each strip to opposite sides of the wound and pull the strips in the direction of the arrows, thus pulling the skin edges toward each other.

wound

Figure 18–11. Alternative type of butterfly bandage. (Using two strips of adhesive tape about 1/4 to 1/2 inch in width and 2 to 3 inches in length).

skin edges separated by 3/8 inch or greater usually need stitches.

    b. Cuts under 1/2 inch long with edges separated by 1/8 inch or less rarely need stitches.

2. Location

    a. Cuts on face, especially the lip or eyelid, need careful attention regardless of size, sometimes by a plastic surgeon. (See Figures 18–12 and 18–13.)

    b. Cuts on the scalp should be seen by a physician. Hair tends to mat in the scab, delaying healing and occasionally leading to infection.

    c. Cuts inside the mouth, though the initial appearance may be bad, usually heal excellently with little or no scar.

3. Age—Only fresh cuts should be stitched (less than four to six hours). Older cuts should be taped loosely with the skin edges apart, so any infection will not be trapped under the skin edges and form an abscess (boil).

Booster Shots

If a child with a small clean cut has had a recent dose of tetanus toxoid, a booster shot will probably not be necessary. However, if the

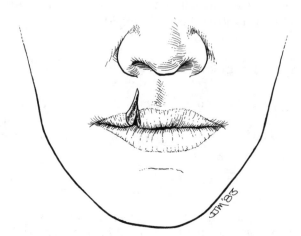

Figure 18–12. Laceration of upper lip.

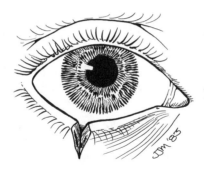

Figure 18–13. Laceration of lower eyelid.

cut is large and dirty, or if the child has not had a recent booster shot, one may be required. This decision should never be made by school personnel; a physician should always be consulted.

PUNCTURE WOUNDS OF THE SKIN

Most puncture wounds of the skin that are caused by small clean objects (pins or paper clips) are minor and need no treatment except cleansing. There is usually no bleeding, and an adhesive bandage should not be applied. (A dab of colored antiseptic may be applied so the child doesn't feel neglected.)

If a child steps on a nail or other sharp object, it is apt to be quite painful and the danger of infection is greater because any germs present will be deposited more deeply into the tissues. The foot should be soaked in warm water for twenty to thirty minutes. Epsom salts or another weak antiseptic may be used. This soaking encourages the wound to remain open and drain as much as possible.

After drying, a loose-fitting covering may be applied so air can enter. If the sole of the foot has been punctured, a small round pad with a hole in the center may be used to relieve pressure. Deciding whether or not to give a booster shot of tetanus toxoid requires the consideration of many factors. Nurses or other school personnel should not make the decision; a physician should be consulted.

A puncture wound caused by the point of a wooden pencil is often seen at school. This cannot cause lead poisoning. The so-called lead in a pencil actually contains no lead; it is compressed graphite, completely inert and nontoxic. It does color the skin and tissue immediately beneath and leaves a small bluish dot which is often permanent; it is actually a small tattoo.

Because of the bluish color, one gets the impression that the pencil tip is broken off under the skin. It is rare that this happens. Unless one can see and feel the actual broken-off point of the pencil sticking up over the skin surface, efforts at removal usually result in greater tissue damage and should not be carried out. Treatment should be limited to cleansing to prevent infection as in any other small puncture wound. If the mark is on the face and is considered unsightly, it may be removed later by plastic surgery.

FRACTURES

Nature of the Condition

A fractured bone is a broken bone; there is no difference. There are numerous different kinds of fractures, but most have one thing in common—they will not heal properly unless put in some type of cast. (See Figures 18–14 through 18–19.)

Symptoms

Pain and swelling and sometimes crookedness can be seen in the fractured arm or leg. In many minor fractures the bones are not out of line, but special treatment such as a cast is usually necessary for proper healing.

During the healing process new bone is built up around the fracture site; this new bone is called *callus*. It often causes a knot or bump that goes away after complete healing.

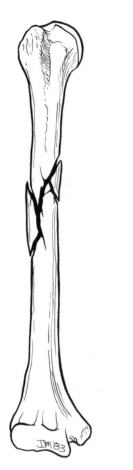

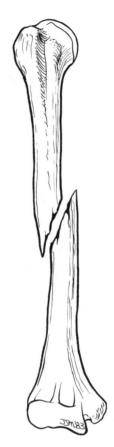

Figure 18–14. Comminuted fracture.   **Figure 18–15.** Oblique fracture.

Treatment and Diagnosis

Any suspected fracture should always be referred to a physician. The diagnosis can only be made with certainty by X-ray. Emergency treatment at school is by splint and sling.

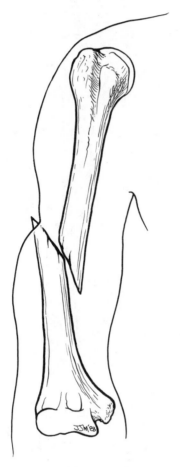

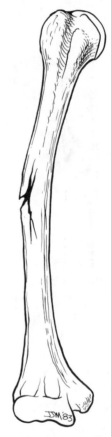

Figure 18–16. Compound fracture.   **Figure 18–17.** Greenstick fracture.

DISLOCATIONS

Nature of the Condition

In school-age children dislocation is most apt to occur in the ball-and-socket joint of the shoulder. (See Figure 18–20.) This may occur following an injury or from throwing a ball too hard. If the elbow, wrist, ankle, knee, or hip becomes dislocated, it usually follows a severe injury and is often accompanied by a fracture.

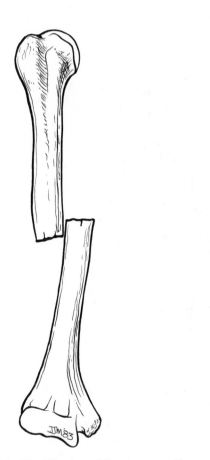 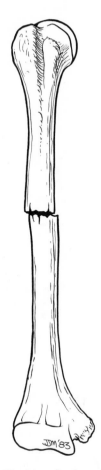

Figure 18–18. Displaced fracture.   **Figure 18–19.** Nondisplaced fracture.

Symptoms

Severe pain and noticeable deformity are always present.

Treatment

After ice application the child should always be referred to a physician, preferably an orthopedic surgeon. Definitive treatment (putting the joint back in place) should never be attempted at school.

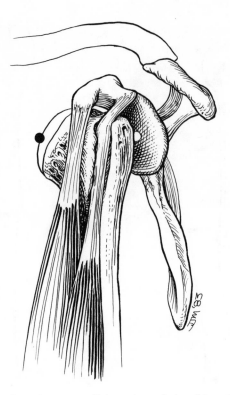

Figure 18–20. Rotation-type dislocation of shoulder. (The shoulder is a ball-and-socket joint. The ball is the upper end of the humerus. The ball's apex is shown by the black dot. The socket is at the lateral plate of the scapula or shoulder blade. When the dislocation is reduced, back in place, the black dot will fit into the white hole.)

This may look easy in the case of a dislocated finger joint, but school nurses, coaches, and athletic trainers should resist the temptation.

Role of the School Nurse

Sprains, strains, fractures, and dislocations are common occurrences at school. Each school should develop a prearranged plan with contacts made in advance at a doctor's office or a hospital emergency room so hasty decisions need not be made in an acute emergency situation.

These procedures should be written and, if possible, posted in the nurse's clinic or the principal's office or both.

Parents must always be notified, but if they are not available, treatment should not be delayed.

ARM AND LEG INJURIES: SPRAIN AND STRAIN

Nature of the Condition

A sprain is a stretching injury of a ligament that does not actually tear it. A strain is a stretching injury of a muscle or tendon that does not actually cause the tendon or muscle to tear or rupture. (See Figure 18–21.)

Either of these injuries can be mild or severe, requiring only a little rest in mild cases or an actual plaster cast in severe cases. They usually occur during athletic contests in secondary school but may also occur during normal childhood play, especially during recess.

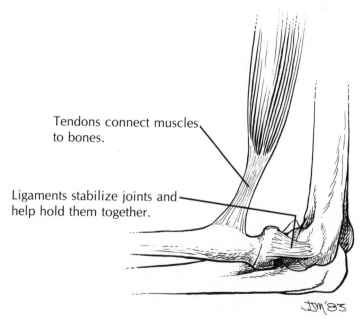

Tendons connect muscles to bones.

Ligaments stabilize joints and help hold them together.

Figure 18–21. Difference between tendon and ligament.

Symptoms

There is pain and swelling, of sudden onset, after twisting the ankle, knee, wrist, elbow, shoulder, hand, or foot.

Treatment

ICE stands for ice, compression, and elevation. Ice can be safely applied directly to the skin, but it is much more comfortable if the ice is first wrapped in a towel. Compression should never be performed by untrained personnel—cutting off the blood supply presents a serious danger. Elevation is often helpful.

Refer to a physician in all but mild cases.

BRUISE

Nature of the Condition

A bruise occurs following sudden impact from a fall or blow by a rock, fist, or other blunt object. The surface of the skin is not broken, but the underlying blood vessels are ruptured and the surrounding tissues are crushed and damaged. In medical jargon, it is called a contusion. A "charley horse" is a bruised muscle.

Symptoms

Pain, redness, and swelling will usually be seen. If the bruise is minor, no redness or swelling will result. At first the blood in the tissues causes reddish discoloration. In a few days the blood gets older and turns bluish-purple and then yellowish-green. This color change demonstrates the age of the bruise. Swelling usually disappears within four days, depending on the severity and location of the bruise. Pain lasts a few minutes in minor bruises, but tenderness persists for days in more severe bruises.

Diagnosis

This is usually obvious from the history and symptoms. However, a child with a disease that causes a delay in blood clotting may be seen with an identical-looking condition and no history of pain or trauma. If the history is reliable, one should examine the child to see if any other bruises are present. If there are, the child should be sent home at the end of the day with a note to the parent.

Treatment

An ice pack will relieve pain. If no ice is readily available, a towel wrung out with cold tap water will help. Commercially available products that produce instant cold packs are available. It would be well to store some of these at each school.

Compression bandages, when indicated, should never be applied by untrained personnel. The danger of cutting off the blood supply is too great. If the injury looks severe, the child should be sent home or to a hospital emergency room with a loose-fitting cold pack.

Elevation of an injured arm with a sling or propping a leg on a chair is helpful.

The procedure outlined above is commonly referred to as ICE treatment, an acronym for ice, compression, and elevation. The same treatment is effective for joint injuries such as sprained ankle or twisted knee, shoulder, or elbow.

Role of the School Nurse

Assess the severity of the bruise. If it is minor yet needs treatment, it may be treated at school; if it is severe, the child should be sent home or to a medical facility.

Be on the alert for nontraumatic discolorations of the skin that resemble bruises; they sometimes occur spontaneously and are often completely painless. If they are on the body or arms, they may have more serious import and, if more than one is seen, parents should be notified. A blood clotting disease may be present.

Warning: Children often have several bruises on their legs, especially between the ankle and knee, and have no knowledge of any injury. These occur during the rough-and-tumble of normal childhood play and need no treatment at all. Also, some adolescent girls (and older women) bruise very easily, such as from a slight bump on the corner of a desk. Bruises limited to the thighs and legs in these individuals need no treatment.

Bruises are one of the most common occurrences a school nurse is called upon to treat. Most children need only a little reassurance, some need ice for relief of pain; few need to be seen by a physician.

Be aware that bruises in different stages of healing on various parts of the body may be warning signals of child abuse.

MUSCLE AND JOINT PAINS—NOT INJURY-RELATED

Nature of the Condition

Pain in the arms and legs occurs in children who have not been injured, much more often in the legs than in the arms, so pain in the arms must be taken more seriously. The pain may be in the muscles or in the joints; the significance and treatment are quite different.

Neck pain (crick in the neck), commonly seen at school, can result from several factors such as sound sleep with the neck in a stressed or twisted position, or excessive cold causing neck muscle tension. Arthritis of a cervical (neck) bone, rare in children, may simulate a crick.

Nontraumatic muscle pain is almost always caused by excessive use during normal childhood play. This is from excessive lactic acid production, a by-product of muscle glycogen metabolism that causes delayed pain by irritation of the muscle. This goes away quickly without intervention. A related condition, growing pains, occurs for the same reason, always in the legs, and it characteristically awakens a child from sleep.

Nontraumatic joint pain may indicate some type of arthritis. It is rare and should be regarded cautiously if it occurs.

Symptoms

Pain is the usual symptom, though redness and swelling may be seen in certain types of arthritis. It is quite common for the pain to occur an hour or two following a play period.

Diagnosis

Differentiation between muscle pain and joint pain is very important; the treatment is different. The best way to tell the difference is by gentle manipulation. Any movement or massage of a diseased joint will usually cause increased pain; gentle massage to a painful, noninjured muscle usually brings relief.

Treatment

Cold applications, by numbing nerve endings and slowing blood circulation, diminish pain and swelling.

Heat applications, by increasing blood circulation, increase tissue metabolism and thus promote healing and return to a normal condition.

Therefore, most traumatic pains are treated with cold, whereas nontraumatic muscle and joint pains are best treated with heat. A heat lamp can provide excellent relief in some cases, but care must be taken not to burn the skin. Hot, wet compresses are equally effective.

Gentle massage can sometimes provide relief, especially if the pain is in the calf muscles. If any manipulation increases the pain, it must be stopped immediately.

Athletes are often advised to exercise a painful muscle to work out the pain. This method should not be used in younger children. At best it should only be used after the cause of the pain is carefully diagnosed by a trained professional.

Role of the School Nurse

If the pain is minor and of short duration, the student can be sent back to class.

If manipulation causes increased pain, stop treatment and allow the child to rest in the clinic. If pain goes away, send the child back to class. If pain persists an hour or more, send the child home.

Emergency evacuation is not necessary unless pain is severe.

BURNS

Figure 18–22 shows the normal layers of skin.

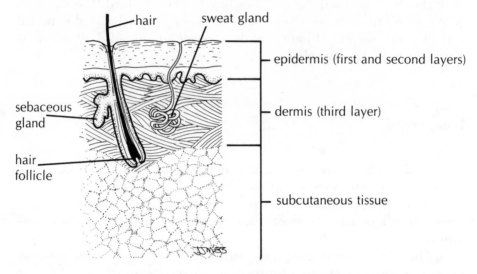

Figure 18–22. Normal layers of skin.

Nature of the Condition and Classification

First degree—redness with no blisters. Mild sunburn is a good example. This involves only the upper part of the first layer.

Second degree—redness with blisters. Severe sunburn or hot liquid are the most common causes. This involves the first and second layers of skin.

Third degree—at least the entire thickness of the skin; may include deeper muscles and even bone in severe burns such as occur in some explosions. The remaining skin tissues may be blanched white or charred black. There are usually no blisters; they have already broken.

Treatment

First degree. Relieve pain with cool compresses or anesthetic ointment (such as benzocain or lanacaine). Nothing else is necessary. Healing always occurs with no scar. As soon as the pain is gone, clean to prevent infection. A tiny burn can have an adehesive bandage applied. The child need not be sent home.

Second degree. Relieve pain with cool compresses, but gently so as not to break any blisters. If the blister can be kept intact, there will be no danger of infection until it eventually breaks, which blisters usually do within several days. A bulky padded bandage should be gently and loosely applied as a first aid measure after equally gentle cleaning with lukewarm water. The child should then see a physician for further treatment. The longer the blister remains intact, the more new skin will grow underneath, so that when the blister does break there will be less likelihood of infection and less pain from raw skin being exposed. A small second-degree burn on the arm or leg can be safely treated at school. It should be washed gently after waiting about ten to fifteen minutes for the pain to subside. Then, after gently patting dry, a small (4 inch by 4 inch) nonsticking gauze flat can be applied and held on with adhesive tape or gauze roller bandage. If in the judgment of the nurse or principal the circumstances are proper and the parent concurs, the child may stay at school but should not go out for recess or gym class for fear of injury to the new burn. Ointments are not harmful, but they moisten and weaken the blister and are conducive to breaking it. The only reason for applying ointment is to relieve pain; cool compresses do this better. Later, if infection is present, antibiotic ointments are necessary but should be prescribed by the physician.

Third degree. These burns are most apt to occur on direct exposure to flames, scalding liquids, or very hot metal. They represent a true medical emergency, not to be treated at school, and should be evacuated to the nearest hospital as quickly as possible. The burns should be covered loosely with a sheet or smooth towel. Ointments should not be applied.

SECTION 19

CLINIC EMERGENCIES

Cardiopulmonary Resuscitation (CPR)
- School Relevance and Role of the School Nurse
- Levels of Training
- Resuscitation Methods
  - —Mouth-to-Mouth Resuscitation
  - —Chest Compression
  - —Back Blows, Heimlich Hug, Finger Sweep of Throat
- Cautions

Temperature Measurement
- Types of Thermometers
- Normal Temperature
- Fever
- Methods of Measurement
- Time of Measurement

Heat-Related Illness
- Nature of the Condition
- Symptoms
- Treatment
- Prevention
- Role of the School Nurse

Fainting
- Nature of the Condition
- Diagnosis and Symptoms
- Treatment and School Relevance

Nosebleed
- Nature of the Condition
- Treatment
- Role of the School Nurse

Food Poisoning
- Diagnosis

Stomachache
- Nature of the Condition
- Symptoms and Treatment

Appendicitis

Headache
- Nature of the Condition
- Treatment and School Relevance

Vomiting
- Nature of the Condition
- Causes
- Role of the School Nurse

Diarrhea
- Nature of the Condition
- Symptoms and Role of the School Nurse
- Treatment

Menstrual Problems
- Nature of the Condition
- Symptoms
- Treatment and School Relevance

Foreign Bodies
- In the Eye
  —Foreign Body
  —Chemical Irritation
- In the Ear
- In the Nose

CARDIOPULMONARY RESUSCITATION (CPR)

School Relevance and Role of the School Nurse

CPR is now the accepted method of lifesaving. Many school districts offer, and some mandate, CPR training to school nurses, secretaries, cafeteria managers, teachers, coaches, athletic trainers, and principals. Athletic trainers and some nurses receive CPR training during their course work leading to certification and licensing.

The school nurse is the person people will instinctively turn to in a medical emergency and therefore is the logical person to be trained in CPR basic life support. However, if the nurse is not on campus daily, it is best to also train someone who is. If the school nurse is selected to be a CPR instructor, it will require a great deal of time out of an already busy schedule and will require the hiring of additional staff.

Levels of Training

The American Heart Association and the American Red Cross have taken the lead in establishing training courses throughout the United States. There are three levels of training and expertise, depending on the time spent in training, teaching, and actually doing CPR.

1. *Resuscitators* are persons trained in basic life support. This requires four to eight hours of training which must be renewed annually.
2. *Instructors* are qualified to teach basic life support. This requires the basic course plus sixteen additional hours of training. In addition, a course must be taught at least twice a year.
3. *Instructor-trainers* are qualified to teach instructors. They must have the same qualifications as instructors and are then selected individually by the program director.

Resuscitation Methods

Detailed CPR instruction is available in many books, booklets, and pamphlets; some are very detailed. This discussion will be limited to the main methods of CPR available and when it should and should not be used.

Mouth-to-Mouth Resuscitation

Mouth-to-mouth resuscitation should only be attempted if there has been a cessation of breathing and a patient is making no respiratory efforts on his or her own. As soon as spontaneous breathing starts, the rescuer should stop so as not to hinder the patient's own breathing efforts.

Chest Compression

When no pulse can be felt in the neck, upper arm, or wrist, proper, intermittent chest compression will keep the blood in circulation. This may keep body cells alive (especially brain cells) until the heart resumes its own spontaneous beat.

Back Blows, Heimlich Hug, Finger Sweep of Throat

Airway obstruction is often caused by a bolus of food, usually a piece of meat. Children may choke on peanuts or popcorn. The patient grasps the front of the throat, cannot speak, turns blue, and rapidly loses consciousness. Coughing is not present.

The Heimlich Hug and sharp blows to the back are both recommended; the Hug to rapidly expel the foreign object, and the back blows to dislodge it if the Hug doesn't work.

If neither of the above works, the finger sweep is a method of thrusting a curled finger into the back of the throat to manually remove the obstructing object.

Note: The Heimlich Maneuver is the only currently accepted method to relieve an obstruction in an adult or child aged one to eight years. Back blows and chest compressions are appropriate for the infant under one year of age. The finger sweep is used on adults—not children.

Cautions

1. All methods of CPR require previous training and practice on a mannequin—never on another person.

2. A person who is coughing should be left alone to cough up whatever is causing the cough.

3. A person who is able to inhale between gags or coughs should be left alone.

4. If the pulse is felt, chest compression should not be attempted.

5. The material in this brief section is not to be considered a substitute for CPR training and complete illustrated handbooks; it is merely a brief summary for school personnel who may have no other immediate resource. An excellent small, practical reference manual is *How to Save a Life Using CPR* by Lindsay R. Curtis, M.D. It is available from H.P. Books, P.O. Box 5367, Tucson, AZ 85703.

TEMPERATURE MEASUREMENT

Types of Thermometers

The *electronic thermometer* is relatively new, very quick, and accurate. It can save time when used for large groups of children. It is expensive—this is its major disadvantage.

The *glass thermometer* is the old standby. It is accurate, inexpensive, and most commonly used. A common misconception is that the thermometer with the long skinny tip is only for oral use and the one with the bulbous tip is only for rectal use. With proper cleansing, they can be used interchangeably.

Recently available are *plastic or paper strips*. Some can be used several times, and some are for single use. They have two disadvantages. If they are used for large groups of children, the total cost can be great. Second, they have not proved to be very accurate. At this time, they are not recommended.

An exception is the new paper strip thermometer, Tempa-DOT.℠ It is considered reliable, needs to be left in the mouth only one minute, and is then discarded. This does away with the need to use plastic sheaths for the reusable glass thermometers. Use of the Tempa-DOT is slightly more expensive, but not excessively so.

The most inaccurate method of all is the old established one of feeling the forehead. Though doctors have urged thermometer use for decades, parents continue to rely on their sense of touch. This is especially risky for children with serious illnesses such as appendicitis or diphtheria which typically begin with a low-grade fever.

Normal Temperature

There is no single level of "normal" body temperature. The traditional glass thermometer has an arrow at 98.6 degrees Fahrenheit because the majority of people in temperate climates have under-tongue temperature readings of about 98.2 to 99 degrees. In actuality, a person's body temperature normally varies from low in the morning to high in the late afternoon and evening. An average healthy person's oral temperature will usually be about 96 to 97 degrees shortly after awakening in the morning and gradually go up to 98 to 99 degrees in the afternoon. Many perfectly normal individuals have an afternoon temperature of 99.6 to 100 degrees, especially in hot summer climates. (see Figure 19–1.)

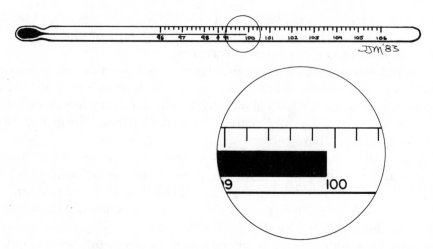

Figure 19–1. Temperature just under 100 degrees

Fever

In order to determine if a child has fever, meaning an abnormal temperature elevation, one must know that child's normal body temperature for the time of the day. Since this is rarely known beforehand, a temperature between 99 and 100 degrees may or may not constitute fever for that individual child. Therefore, unless a child has some other symptoms of illness, doctors are apt to regard an oral temperature of 100 degrees or less as only a possible sign of illness and suggest that the child be watched closely for further symptoms.

Temperature readings over 100 degrees usually indicate some type of infection, though there are a small number of normal individuals with no illness at all, even while having a temperature of 100 to 100.6 degrees. Readings of 101 degrees and over are always abnormal and are to be considered as fever.

Methods of Measurement

The usual methods of temperature measurement are oral, rectal, and axillary (armpit). The first two are more reliable; the axillary temperature varies more with changes in air temperature.

There is an old rule of thumb which states that at any given time the rectal temperature is one degree higher than the oral and the axillary is one degree lower than the oral. This is not accurate. Generally speaking, the rectal temperature is somewhat higher than the oral and the axillary is lower, but it is practically never exactly one degree and there are times when they are the same. Therefore, it is incorrect to think that a rectal temperature of 100 degrees is always normal. The level of the body temperature is only one of several indicators of disease. When recording or reporting temperature, one should always state the actual thermometer reading and in what part of the body it was measured.

Time of Measurement

The number of minutes the thermometer should be left in place varies with the type of thermometer used, but most instructional pamphlets suggest leaving it in place about three minutes; this is usually longer than necessary. In most cases, the thermometer will reach its peak in one minute. It is easy enough to take the thermometer out after one minute, read it, reinsert it, and read it after another minute. The reading will be the same or 0.2 to 0.4 degree higher. Using this method, the school nurse or clinic aide learns how long the thermometer must be left in place and saves time and some discomfort for the child.

Factors causing misleading temperature readings include:

1. Excessive environmental heat and humidity
2. Excessive exposure to cold
3. Excessive physical exercise
4. Decreased air circulation
5. Recent eating or drinking of hot or cold foods
6. A child sneaking the thermometer under the hot water faucet because he or she wants to go home

HEAT-RELATED ILLNESS

Nature of the Condition

There are four types of adverse physical reactions to excess heat and humidity. The higher the humidity, the more dangerous is a high air temperature because of decreased evaporation of body sweat. Exercise causes increased sweating and body metabolism which leads to greater loss of body water and electrolytes (sodium, potassium, etc.). If these losses are severe, the adverse reactions may vary from simple fainting to fatal heat stroke. This can occur indoors and in climates that are not excessively hot.

Symptoms

1. *Heat syncope.* This is simple fainting or near fainting caused by overheating. It begins with dizziness, usually while the student is standing or running. The blood pressure goes down, and the body

(rectal) temperature is high—103 to 105 degrees Fahrenheit. The skin is usually moist.

2. *Heat cramps.* Tightening, cramps, and spasm of active muscles occur, usually during intense, prolonged exercise in hot weather. There is no loss of consciousness. This is associated with low body sodium.

3. *Heat exhaustion.* The early symptoms are dizziness, weakness, exhaustions, nausea, and vomiting. The student may become irrational and belligerent. There may be associated muscle cramps. The rectal temperature is high. The skin is flushed and usually moist, but in extreme cases it can be dry. If the symptoms continue, partial or complete unconsciousness may ensue and lead to heat stroke.

4. *Heat stroke.* This is an acute medical emergency with extremely high fever, 106 to 108 degrees Fahrenheit, disorientation, twitching, seizures, and coma. The skin is hot and dry.

Heat-related illnesses are usually not seen as clearly separate entities; they often merge into each other, especially if proper treatment is delayed. For example, there may be doubt about heat exhaustion versus impending heat stroke. Whenever there is doubt, always suspect the worst.

Treatment

Heat syncope, heat cramps, and heat exhaustion are all treated by rest, placement in a cool, shaded area, replacement of water by drinking, and cooling of the skin with cold water and/or a fan. This is usually sufficient.

Heavy clothing should be loosened or removed, and resumption of exercise should be delayed for at least two to three hours.

Children who experience more severe symptoms such as irrationality or partial loss of consciousness should be evaluated by their physician.

If heat stroke occurs, oral fluids can rarely be swallowed. Rapid evacuation to a medical emergency room is mandatory but at the same time the skin should be cooled with water, ice, and/or a fan. If available, oxygen should be given.

Prevention

All heat-related illness is preventable if proper measures are taken.

1. Exercise preconditioning, heat acclimatization, and water replacement are the most important factors.
2. Lightweight, loose, cool clothing should be worn.
3. Athletes are at special risk and occasionally require enforced extra water intake.
4. Cool or cold water should be available, since it is absorbed more quickly from the stomach.
5. Salt and calcium tablets are of no benefit. If enough water is drunk, the body automatically conserves salt and calcium, so it is not necessary to give tablets.
6. Commercial electrolyte solutions are not harmful and may be used if desired. They are no more effective than water.
7. Students who sweat a lot should salt their food more liberally.
8. Predisposing conditions that make a child more likely to develop heat illness are as follows:
   a. Cystic fibrosis
   b. Vomiting or diarrhea
   c. Fever from any cause, even an immunization
   d. Obesity
   e. Voluntary water restriction
   f. Poor acclimatization
   g. Prior heat-related illness

Role of the School Nurse

If no qualified athletic trainers are available, the school nurse's expertise may be lifesaving. The following factors are to be considered:

1. Plenty of cool water should be available to students during all game and practice sessions.
2. Athletes who lose more than 3 percent of their body weight (about 5 to 7 pounds for a 200-pound athlete) because of sweat

loss during a practice session, are at special risk. An accurate scale should be available.

3. Athletic personnel should be alerted to the possible dangers of excess salt tablets causing high-sodium dehydration. High water intake is much more efficient in maintaining good fluid and electrolyte balance.

4. All personnel should be cautioned about the dangers of voluntary water deprivation to produce weight loss, especially in athletes.

5. The Sports Medicine Guide and the School Health Guide, both published by the American Academy of Pediatrics, contain additional useful information. They can be ordered from P.O. Box 927, Elk Grove Village, IL 60009.

FAINTING

Nature of the Condition

Fainting can occur for a variety of reasons, including weakness, hunger, strong emotional reactions, severe pain, or onset of an illness. Some individuals are more prone to faint than others. For unknown reasons, it is more common in girls.

Fainting usually is associated with a sudden decrease in blood supply to the brain and may or may not be associated with low blood pressure and slow pulse. Sudden change in position, especially from a lying or sitting to a standing position, can cause dizziness or even fainting.

Diagnosis and Symptoms

Fainting can occur for a variety of reasons, including weakness, simple fainting spell there are usually no twitching movements of the arms and legs. If there is any twitching, a physician will be required to rule out epilepsy.

Treatment and School Relevance

1. Place the head on the same level with or lower than the chest. If dizziness occurs while sitting in a chair, lower the head between the knees. A child who has fainted and is lying on the floor should remain there until recovery.

2. Check pulse and respiration. If they are normal, one can be reassured that the child will soon recover.

3. Blood pressure should be measured if possible. If the pressure is not excessively low (below 90/60), the fainting spell is less likely to be serious.

4. Many school nurses and teachers know which children in school are habitual fainters. When a child faints who has never fainted before, one must be cautious and suspect more serious causes.

5. Attempts to awaken the child do not help; they are an expression of anxiety on the part of the adult. It is better to observe the child for a short time and check the blood pressure, pulse, and respiration. If the child moves or groans, it is an indication that he or she is not deeply unconscious. If signs point to deepening unconsciousness, evacuate to a hospital or doctor's office.

NOSEBLEED

Nature of the Condition

Nosebleeds are most common in children four to ten years, mostly in boys. Children with colds or nasal allergies have more nosebleeds, not only because the lining of the nose is more irritated, but because they pick more and blow harder.

Since more colds occur in winter, more nosebleeds occur then. However, vigorous exercise in hot weather can also bring on nosebleeds in children without colds. Repeated nosebleeds in the same child are common.

Some older girls get nosebleeds each time they menstruate; this is rare. It is called "vicarious menstruation."

Treatment

The child should be in a sitting position with the upper body tilted forward so the blood does not run back down the throat and be swallowed. For comfort, the forehead can rest against the wall. Excess blood irritates the stomach and causes vomiting. Some children have nosebleeds while asleep and the first the parent knows about it is when the child vomits blood on awakening.

Since most nosebleeds are due to tiny ruptured blood vessels near the tip of the nose on the inner wall (the nasal septum), the best treatment is firm pressure pinching the end of the nose shut. Usually it takes five minutes to stop all bleeding (time it by the clock). Sometimes fifteen minutes is necessary. If you can determine that the blood is coming from one side only, you need to apply only pressure against that side.

After the bleeding stops, have the child rest in the school clinic for fifteen or twenty minutes before going back to class. Play during recess or PC should be skipped for that day.

Always notify the parents. Very few children with nosebleeds need to be referred to the doctor.

There are three main reasons for referral:

1. There is bleeding from other parts of the body—blood spots under the skin, blood in the urine, etc.
2. The bleeding occurs almost daily.
3. The bleeding won't stop.

If the bleeding doesn't stop with pressure, and the child cannot be taken to an emergency room right away, a tight packing can be put in the nose. Be careful not to pack past the tip of the nose. This is safe if done properly, usually with gauze from a roller-bandage and blunt forceps. This will stop the bleeding in most cases.

Folk Remedies: Common folk remedies use a key or ice pack on the back of the neck, or a rolled up piece of paper under the upper lip. While none of these remedies do any harm, be sure to compress the tip of the nose at the same time.

Role of the School Nurse

The child should be excused from recess or other outdoor physical activity for that day only. Parents should be notified. Medical referral is necessary only in severe nosebleeds (more than fifteen minutes), frequently recurring nosebleeds, or bleeding in other body areas.

FOOD POISONING

Diagnosis

Fever is rarely present, though it may occur.

Check with the school medical consultant to see if there is an epidemic of gastrointestinal disease in the community or at other schools. Schools that do not have an individual consultant can call the local health department.

Since the symptoms of food poisoning (vomiting, stomachache, and diarrhea) almost always occur within twenty-four hours of ingestion of the contaminated food, it is recommended that every school cafeteria routinely save, in the refrigerator, for twenty-four hours, a tray of food from every meal every day. If an outbreak occurs, this food can then be analyzed for toxic bacteria.

STOMACHACHE

Nature of the Condition

All children have stomachaches occasionally. The causes are numerous. It is by far the most common childhood complaint, and most of the time the condition is minor, needs no special treatment, and goes away by itself. Stomachaches can also be caused by emotional distress. This does not mean the child is emotionally disturbed; it is simply his or her particular reaction to stress. Other children may react to stress with a headache. One of the most common causes of stomachache is *mesenteric adenitis*. This means swelling of the lymph nodes in the abdomen, a temporary condition that may accompany many common childhood diseases, such as the common cold, influenza, or chicken pox.

Emotional causes of stomachache are extremely varied. Some of the more common are:

1. School academic failure
2. Not liking the teacher (or vice versa)
3. Being harassed by a bully on the playground or around school
4. Parental or sibling anxiety, child abuse, or other home problems
5. School phobia

Though some older children can talk about problems of this nature, it is usually unrealistic to expect it of younger children.

Symptoms and Treatment

1. *Fever.* This can only be determined by using a thermometer and indicates an organic cause (as opposed to emotional). It is usually an indication for sending the child home. A child with a stomachache without fever could possibly have something serious, but it is much less likely.

2. *Facial expression.* A child who complains of a stomachache, looks alert, does not seem worried, or does not frown as if in pain, usually does not have a serious condition. Such a child needs to rest in the school clinic for a while, and if no fever is present and the pain is gone in ten or fifteen minutes, it is safe to send him or her back to class. Suggest that the child come back later if his or her stomach starts to hurt again.

3. *Vomiting or diarrhea.* If either of these symptoms is present, the child usually has a disease that is contagious, and he or she should be sent home.

4. *Position of comfort.* If the child is just as comfortable sitting in a chair as lying on a cot, it usually indicates a less serious type of stomachache.

5. *Progression of pain.* In the more serious stomachaches, the pain usually gets worse after an hour or two; in the less serious, the pain usually diminishes within the first hour after onset.

APPENDICITIS

When a child with a stomachache comes to the clinic, school personnel are concerned because appendicitis, if left untreated, can progress rapidly and lead to rupture with *peritonitis* (infection of the entire abdominal cavity), an extremely serious disease. While no school nurse or other school person should take the responsibility for making such a diagnosis, there are certain symptoms that should make one suspicious.

1. *Fever.* Early in the course of appendicitis the fever is low, 99.6 to 101 degrees Fahrenheit in most cases. For this reason it is most important to use a thermometer. It is impossible to detect a fever of 100 degrees by feeling a child's forehead.

2. *Location and progression of pain.* The pain characteristically begins in the pit of the stomach—in the center and just below the ribs—and as it increases in severity, it gradually moves to the lower right, halfway between the navel and the groin. The pain slowly but surely gets worse. This is an important symptom, characteristic of appendicitis. The speed of progression varies a great deal—the younger the child, the faster. In general, however, in a first to fifth grade child (ages six to eleven), the pain that begins in the pit of the stomach will have moved down to the lower right quadrant of the abdomen within two to six hours. In a three-year-old, progress is often faster.

3. *Facial expression.* The child with appendicitis does not come into the clinic smiling; he or she usually looks uncomfortable.

4. *Position of comfort.* In appendicitis, the child would rather lie down than sit up, often on the left side with the right leg drawn up.

5. *Other findings.* These include constipation, loss of appetite, and abdominal tenderness to pressure, but these symptoms are best evaluated by a physician. If appendicitis is suspected, the parents should be called and the child should be taken to the doctor immediately.

HEADACHE

Nature of the Condition

Headache is a common symptom of emotional anxiety as well as organic disease. One must assess many of the same factors seen in children with stomachaches. Fever and facial expression have the same import. A happy child without a fever does not in all likehood have a serious headache.

Some physicians feel that a child who misses breakfast may get a headache from hunger. Others do not agree. In any case, it never hurts to offer a child with a headache something to eat—if the child is hungry. Juice, milk, biscuits, or cookies in small amounts will do no harm. If the child is not hungry, it is better not to eat because it may precipitate vomiting.

The following accompanying symptoms are important warning signs and, if present, the child should be sent home:

1. Dizziness
2. Blurred vision
3. Fainting
4. Fever
5. Drowsiness
6. Nausea/vomiting
7. Persistence for an hour or more

Treatment and School Relevance

A short rest in the clinic is usually all that is necessary. However, many children have minor headaches fairly often, and parents will ask the school nurse or principal to give the child Tylenol™ whenever he or she complains of a headache. Parents, and sometimes even school personnel, are often unaware that all nurses, including school nurses, are prohibited by law from giving any medication—prescription or nonprescription—that is not ordered by a licensed physician. School nurses often fear action by their state licensing agency (loss of license) as well as later litigation by parents. Parents, on the other hand, simply cannot understand why a school nurse cannot do such a simple thing as give a child acetaminophen (Tylenol℗) or aspirin (see section on Reye Syndrome), or other nonprescription medication for an occasional headache. If the parent gets a note from the physician authorizing the school nurse (or other delegated personnel) to administer the medicine, and this note is also signed by the parent, the school authorities have sufficient legal protection. Otherwise, the school physician consultant can discuss each individual case with the school nurse and give the necessary medical order.

VOMITING

Nature of the Condition

Nausea and vomiting are very common childhood symptoms. Almost any illness can cause a child to vomit. At school the nurse must decide whether this symptom is the result of a disease for which the parent must be called and the child sent home, or whether to have the child lie down in the clinic for ten to twenty minutes.

Causes

1. *Minor childhood illnesses.* There are literally hundreds of bacteria and viruses that cause gastrointestinal upsets in children, often associated with fever.

2. *Emotional anxiety.*

3. *Food poisoning.* Though this is often of primary concern in a school that serves meals, it is actually a rare occurrence. However, many children vomiting on the same day should raise the suspicion that they ate spoiled or contaminated food from the school cafeteria. There are many bacteria that contaminate food and many requirements that school cafeterias follow to prevent outbreaks. One of the best ways to avoid risks is to subscribe to *Morbidity and Mortality Weekly Reports* and the *FDA Consumer* (see Section 1.)

Role of the School Nurse

One episode of vomiting does not necessarily mean the child needs to see a doctor—or even to go home. Vomiting one time can be from too much exercise in the hot sun, strong emotional factors (fear, anxiety, etc.), or other causes which soon pass.

Fever, as measured by the thermometer, is probably the most important factor to consider in assessment. When present, send the child home.

Facial expression, an important sign, should be assessed after a five- to ten-minute wait. If there is continued or increased discomfort, send the child home.

After the child vomits once, the school nurse should allow him or her to lie down in the clinic, take the temperature, and see how the child feels in ten to twenty minutes. Then a decision should be made about whether to call the parents.

Blood in the vomitus is not necessarily a serious sign. On vomiting, the stomach muscles contract very tightly and frequently cause some of the smaller blood vessels to rupture. Therefore, many children who vomit, especially if they retch hard, will have some bloody streaks of mucus mixed with their stomach contents. The seriousness of the bleeding can be judged entirely by the amount of blood one sees. A few streaks should cause no alarm. Anything more than this, especially tablespoon quantities of blood, should be cause for emergency measures. Obviously, nothing can be done at school; arrangements should be made to transport the child to the nearest emergency room immediately, and the parents should be notified, in that order.

DIARRHEA

Nature of the Condition

Many of the same minor childhood diseases that cause vomiting can cause diarrhea in younger babies. However, school-age children who develop diarrhea usually have a specific intestinal disease. Many are caused by viruses, are minor, and are of short duration. Roughly half of the children with mild diarrhea have low-grade fever. This type of mild diarrhea usually lasts two or three days and goes away by itself.

Some children develop more severe diarrhea with higher fever. These children are likely to have more stomachache from intestinal cramping and will usually have most severe cramping pain just before another bowel movement. After the bowel movement the pain will diminish for a while. It is rare for children with diarrhea to have only one loose stool and stop; they usually have more.

The contagiousness of any given case of diarrhea depends entirely on the cause. However, most cases are contagious, and appropriate precautions should be taken.

Symptoms and Role of the School Nurse

1. *Fever.* Children with mild diarrhea may have none at all; severe cases usually have more. When present, send the child home.
2. *Soiling of clothes at school.* This causes a child great distress. If facilities are available, the child should be cleaned up; if not, he or she should be helped home as quickly as possible.
3. *Stomachache*
4. *Loss of appetite*

Treatment

Kaopectate is one of the few medicines available that has no adverse side effects. It can be obtained over the counter and can be given in perfect safety according to directions on the bottle.

A child with diarrhea should not be urged to eat, but light foods in small quantities are all right if the child is hungry. To prevent dehydration and to maintain the flow of urine, liquids are important and should be urged.

Most cases are mild and get well without treatment. Severe cases with fever and cramps should be referred to a physician.

MENSTRUAL PROBLEMS

Nature of the Condition

The medical problems associated with menstruation fall under the following three categories:

1. Pain
2. Excessive bleeding
3. Unexpected bleeding

Symptoms

Excessive menstrual pain—dysmenorrhea, is common in school-age girls. It begins one to three years after the menarche (onset of menstruation) and practically always disappears after the birth of the first child. The pain can be severe and accompanied by vomiting, headache, and backache. A day or two of school may be missed each month.

Excessive bleeding means either more frequent than approximately once a month, or once a month but excessive in amount.

Normal menstruation does not occur more often than twenty-one days from the first day of one period to the first day of the next, the bleeding does not last more than six days, and not more than six well-soaked pads are used every twenty-four hours.

Unexpected bleeding can be caused by unexpected menarche or unexpected onset of a period in a previously menstruating girl.

Treatment and School Relevance

1. Have the girl lie down in school clinic.
2. Give acetaminophen, not aspirin. (Follow state and school rules.) Girls do not have to suffer each month from cramps as they used to. There are safe medications such as Advil or

Nuprin that are helpful in preventing dysmenorrhea. Suggest that the student have her mother consult a physician for advice.

3. This is a perfect opportunity to establish rapport which will make the school nurse a primary resource adult for future questions relating to sex. Do not assume that the student knows what is happening to her, how to use pads, or the danger of toxic shock syndrome from using tampons.

4. Suggest that she keep a calendar so her periods will not catch her unprepared.

5. If pain continues, refer to physician.

6. Send her home if pain is severe. (Follow state and school rules.)

7. Refer her to a physician if pain continues.

FOREIGN BODIES

In the Eye

A speck of dirt, a cinder, or another tiny foreign object that suddenly lodges in the eye will cause sudden pain and excessive tearing. Chemicals or other liquid irritants can cause lasting damage and need rapid special treatment. (Cuts or bruises of the eye are discussed in Section 18.)

Foreign Body

If the child is cooperative and quiet, the lid can be pulled down and away from the eyeball, as shown in Figures 19–2 and 19–3. This may loosen the foreign body and allow tears to wash it away. If the object is easy to see resting on the lid (not on the eyeball), it can be safely removed with a cotton-tipped applicator.

In all other circumstances the child should be encouraged to blink frequently and not to rub the eye. If the foreign body is not gone in a few minutes, an eye specialist should be consulted. If the child is sent to an eye specialist, the affected eye should be covered with a 2 inch by 2 inch gauze flat held in place with criss-crossed adhesive strips.

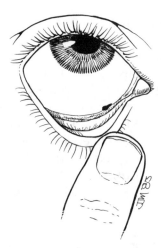

Figure 19–2. Foreign body in lower lid

Chemical Irritation

Acid or alkaline solutions in the eye must be washed out immediately with copious amounts of plain tap water. Do not waste time searching for special neutralizing solutions. It is important to use water in large volume, *not* to squirt it into the eye in a small jet stream with rapid force. Ideally, the child should be lying down, the eyelids should be held wide open, and a gentle stream of cool water about 1/4 to

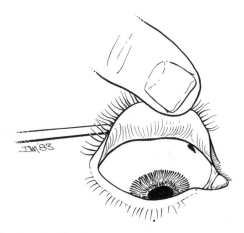

Figure 19–3. Foreign body in upper lid. (Lid is rolled back over a cotton swab.)

1/2 inch in diameter should be allowed to run into the eye at the inner corner and out of the outer corner, so the head must be slightly tilted toward the side of the affected eye. (See Figure 19–4.)

In any emergency of this nature, never be concerned about a wet bed, floor, or clothes. The above described physical apparatus is rarely available at a school. As a substitute, a team of three people can help calm the child and hold the lids open, slowly pour a glass of water into the inner corner of the eye, and keep a second glass of water constantly filled so flushing is uninterrupted. Most acid and alkaline solutions are sticky; the water should run for fifteen to thirty minutes.

While the eye is being flushed without interruption, a phone call to the eye specialist will help make a judgment as to how long to continue irrigation before taking the child to the eye doctor. If the irrigation is not proceeding smoothly and the water is not flushing the

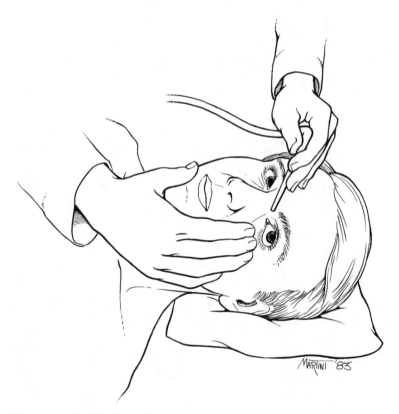

Figure 19–4. Flushing chemical irritant from eye. (Upper lid must be held up also.)

eyeball, go to the doctor sooner. Tape a 4 inch by 4 inch gauze flat over the eye for the trip to the doctor.

In the Ear

Children often push erasers, paper wads, beans, or other objects into their ears. (See Figure 19–5.) This usually causes no pain, so the child doesn't report it. It is discovered during a later routine physical checkup.

Occasionally an insect will fly into the ear. The buzzing and movement cause intense discomfort while the insect is alive. Lidocaine drops (a local anesthetic), if available, work well to kill insects. Do not use mineral oil—it causes the inset to swell and makes it harder to remove later.

Nurses or other school personnel should never try to remove any foreign object from the ear unless it is sticking out and can be easily grasped with the fingers or forceps. Foreign objects in the ear are quite difficult to get out. Without the proper equipment, special technique, and good lighting, the object will be pushed in farther.

Foreign bodies in the ear are not emergency conditions but should be referred to a physician as soon as feasible.

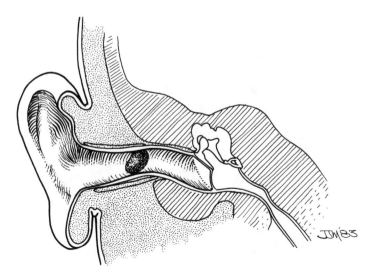

Figure 19–5. Foreign body in ear.

In the Nose

Children push the same objects into their noses as they do into their ears. (See Figure 19–6.) There is no pain, and often parents or school personnel are not told by the child. However, since the nose is always moist, infection ensues and causes a foul-smelling nasal discharge from only one nostril. Nasal discharge from a common cold, sinus, or allergy is seen on both sides and rarely is associated with an odor.

Exactly the same warnings apply as for foreign bodies in the ear. Occasionally a child will report a foreign body in the nose. Unless it is sticking out, any attempts to remove it will just push it in farther.

Two removal methods have recently been described in medical journals:

1. Blow into the mouth while holding unobstructed nostril shut. The nurse can explain the procedure to the parent.
2. Strong but careful suction with a rubber catheter: This is usually only feasible in an emergency room or doctor's office.

This is not an emergency condition, but the child should be referred to a physician as soon as feasible.

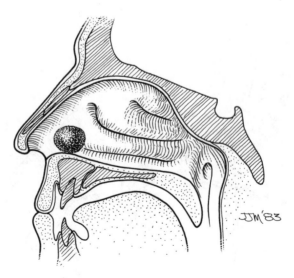

Figure 19–6. Foreign body in nose.

SECTION 20

SEVERE PHYSICAL DISABILITIES

Public Law 94-142

Mainstreaming
- School Relevance and Role of the School Nurse
  —Is the Disease Progressive; Is It Getting Worse?

Special Nursing Procedures
- Clean Intermittent Catheterization (CIC)
- Pharyngeal and Nasopharyngeal Suctioning
- Colostomy, Ileostomy, Nephrostomy, and Other Ostomy Bags
- Tracheostomy
- Gastrostomy and Tube Feeding

Occupational and Physical Therapy in the School System
- Historical Introduction
- Children on the Borderline
- Role of the School Nurse
- Relation to Physician
- Legal Aspects

Students with Special Health Needs
- Least Restrictive Environment

Spina Bifida
- Nature of the Condition
- Diagnosis and Symptoms

337

- Treatment
- School Relevance and Role of the School Nurse
  —Skin of the Lower Back
  —Bowel Care
  —Bladder Care
  —Care of the Legs, Braces, and Crutches
  —Observation of Head Size
  —Class Placement and Learning Problems
  —Special Problems at Adolescence

Mental Retardation
- Nature of the Condition
  —High-Level
  —Low-Level
- Diagnosis and Symptoms
  —High-Level
  —Low-Level
- Treatment
  —High-Level
  —Low-Level

PUBLIC LAW 94-142

Since the passage in 1975 of Public Law (PL) 94-142, Education for All Handicapped Children, there has been a concerted effort to include disabled children in the regular school system, public and private. School systems along with groups outside the school system—parents, doctors, cerebral palsy associations, lawyers, physiotherapists, occupational therapists, and others—have contributed to the effort.

In past years, most parents of children with severe physical disabilities were advised to keep their children home, keep them clean, and were not encouraged to teach them.

Most children with cerebral palsy were regarded by parents and doctors alike as mentally retarded as well. With experience and better understanding, it has become apparent that various kinds of education and training are indeed beneficial. There is no longer any doubt that most disabled children belong in a school setting. They are happier, and they make greater advances in self-help and other skills than when they stay home. Many schools have proved successful in providing education for disabled children from kindergarten through high school, graduating many who become partially or fully independent adults.

MAINSTREAMING

Most disabled children manage fairly well in a regular mainstream class. However, because of pressures that have arisen since passage of PL 94-142, some severely disabled children are being placed in regular mainstream classes. Such a child may have the same hopes, fears, disappointments, and desires for acceptance as other children of that age, even though he or she is unable to communicate or play with peers. It is a developmental period during which even normal children have little insight into themselves or the distresses of others. Feelings of empathy come later in life, beginning in preadolescence and coming to fruition in late adolescence. Therefore, the severely disabled child needs support and protection from peers.

Each case is individual, and placement should be based on what is best for the child, not on an educational or psychological philosophy developed by distant, so-called experts. The most difficult cases to decide are those in which physical handicap is severe and intellectual function is normal or superior. A recently published book, written by a profoundly disabled person, is recommended for insight into the range of potential found in this group. (See *Under the Eye of the Clock*, by Christopher Nolan, New York: St. Martin's, 1988.)

Tentative trials can determine whether or not the child is ready for mainstreaming in a regular or a special class on a regular campus. The school nurse should be aware that the desire of the parents that their children be as near normal as possible is strong, and there may be disagreement over the child's placement. With nursing expertise and physician liaison, the school nurse has valuable input to help parents and school personnel decide on proper class placement.

School Relevance and Role of the School Nurse

Is the child contagious? (See Section 9.) Babies born with congenital herpes simplex or congenital rubella (German measles) may be severely mentally retarded and may be contagious for varying periods of time. The virus can be found in various body secretions, including saliva.

Babies with congenital rubella often shed virus for weeks or months, but never years. By the age of three years, they are no longer contagious. If teachers or other school personnel must be near younger children with rubella, they might contract the disease. Therefore, they should be tested for susceptibility (a simple blood test) and immunized with rubella vaccine if necessary. This is especially true if the teacher is of childbearing age; rubella infection in the early months of pregnancy can lead to serious birth defects.

It takes about six weeks for the teacher to develop immunity after immunization. If a very young (under one-year-old) rubella baby is to be admitted to school, ample time must be allowed for all necessary school personnel to develop immunity after receiving the vaccine.

Pregnant women or women who could become pregnant within six weeks are cautioned not to receive the vaccine. It is a live virus vaccine, and there is a possibility of the virus being transmitted to the fetus and causing congenital rubella. A serious dilemma may arise if the school has a special education program that admits very young babies and some of the teachers in that building are susceptible to rubella and may be pregnant or become pregnant. The solution to this dilemma is administrative. Homebound programs or teacher transfers are two options.

Herpes simplex virus may infect a fetus during pregnancy and cause severe brain damage. Some of these infants live for many years with severe physical and mental retardation, and some will be enrolled in public schools. If they have fever blisters around their mouths and noses, they are just as contagious as any normal child with the fever blisters of herpes simplex. However, since they must be handled more and since they often drool, the opportunity for spread of the virus is greater. Therefore, handwashing is more important. Also, the school nurse should set up certain techniques, procedures, and routines similar to those used in hospital contagious disease wards but adapted to school use.

The herpes virus in children with brain damage caused by congenital herpes acts in the same way as it does in normal children who contract herpes from friends. It lies dormant in the body and is only contagious when it becomes manifest as the familiar cold sore or fever blister seen around the mouth or nose.

Is the Disease Progressive; Is It Getting Worse?

The majority of children with severe mental deficiency have nonprogressive disease. The damage to the brain was suffered long before, and the infection or trauma is no longer present, although complications such as pneumonia and bed sores occur frequently and often lead to early death.

There are, however, rare diseases of the brain that lead to progressive brain damage. These diseases are often fatal. They are discussed in Section 7 under the heading "Progressive Diseases of the Nervous System." They are rarely, if ever, contagious. The role of the school nurse is simply to offer supportive nursing care as long as the child remains in school.

SPECIAL NURSING PROCEDURES

Increasingly, nursing procedures previously performed only in hospitals are now being done by school nurses. Some school districts are having problems adjusting to this requirement; others have seen it as an opportunity to help normalize the student's life. The procedures now being performed include:

- bladder catheterization
- gastrostomy, nasogastric, or orogastric tube feeding
- ileostomy or colostomy bag changes and care
- nephrostomy bag changes and care
- tracheostomy care
- pharyngeal and nasopharyngeal suctioning
- postural drainage with chest massage
- peritoneal dialysis

All of these procedures are described in step-by-step detail in many nursing textbooks and are familiar to professional nurses. Therefore, I will discuss the parts of each procedure that are particularly related to doing them in school, as opposed to home or hospital.

If the school nurse has not performed the particular procedure for many years, brush-up instructions from another nurse or doctor who does the procedure regularly should be arranged. (One of my frequent duties is to give short refresher courses to health service personnel who need to do clean intermittent bladder catheterization.)

Clean Intermittent Catheterization (CIC)

This special procedure is now commonly carried out at school, frequently for children with spina bifida with bladder paralysis, to keep the bladder empty so stagnant urine will not cause an infection.

- Clean=The catheter need not be sterilized, only clean.
- Intermittent=The catheter need not be left in the bladder (indwelling), but merely inserted, the urine in the bladder drained, and the catheter withdrawn.

The usual frequency of catheterization is four times day, about four to six hours apart. On this schedule, it should be done at school between 11:00 A.M. and 1:00 P.M. The parent should do it at home at 7:00 A.M., at 4:00 or 5:00 P.M., and at bedtime. On occasion, a doctor or parent will request that the child be catheterized twice a day at school, for nonmedical reasons, such as the parent leaving early for work. In these cases, each school district will have to make an administrative decision; once a day at school is sufficient for the child's medical needs.

The school should provide a good light and a high, steady, padded table, especially necessary for catheterizing little girls. The urethral orifice, when the labia are separated, may look like one of the many tiny folds in the circumvaginal area and without good light and a firm, non-wiggly surface, it is easy to insert the catheter tip into the vagina.

The catheters, usually plastic and disposable, may be used several times until they are no longer soft and pliable. Some parents prefer to use a new catheter each day and others will not bring a new catheter until the nurse requests it. After each use, the catheter should be cleaned with soap and water. Because they are so small, it may be necessary to force water through with a hypodermic syringe to clean the inside. They may be stored in their original paper container until the next use.

The amount of urine recovered from each child will vary from 5–10 cc to 1–2 ounces. Usually, the free end of the catheter drains into an emesis basin or other suitable container. If the nurse knows from experience that only 5–10 cc of urine will emerge, the catheter can drain on the diaper, which is usually wet and must be changed anyway.

This special procedure, clean intermittent catheterization, is simple (easier to do than giving a shot). Almost all parents can be trained in the technique in a short time. Health aides can easily be trained to do it, but since the parent is not present, it is legally risky. In my district, it is performed only by registered school nurses.

The form, "Special Procedure for Clean Intermittent Catheterization (CIC)," may be included in the school nurses' procedure book.

SPECIAL PROCEDURE FOR CLEAN INTERMITTENT CATHETERIZATION (CIC)

I. INTRODUCTION

CIC is a clean (not sterile) procedure that is normally done three or four times a day to empty the bladder. Its aim is to maintain an infection-free urinary tract as well as socially-accepted dryness. It is done by the school nurse for children with spina bifida until they are able to do it for themselves. It is an activity of daily living for many children with spina bifida and self-catheterization should be learned as soon as possible. The campus nurse will also serve as liaison between home, school, and health community in matters related to the student's other medical and health care needs.

(continued)

II. PROGRAM GOALS

A. Decrease the occurrence of urinary tract infection
B. Regular and frequent emptying of the bladder at planned times
C. If possible, eliminate the need for diapers
D. Prevent overstretching of the bladder and preserve the muscle tone of the bladder wall
E. Have child take care of his/her bladder program completely and independently as soon as possible
F. Allow the child normal physical, social and emotional functioning, free from worry about bladder accidents, thus preserving his/her self respect

III. THE FOLLOWING GUIDELINES ARE RECOMMENDED FOR THE CAMPUS NURSE IN MANAGEMENT OF THE STUDENT REQUIRING CIC

A. Conduct a parent conference to ascertain current health status of student and to obtain approval to confer with other health care professionals about the student's health needs.
B. Obtain current recommendations from the student's doctor.
C. Design and assist with implementation of the individual health management plan for the student as part of the student's individual education plan (IEP).

IV. GUIDELINES FOR PERFORMING CIC

A. Equipment needed
   1. Soap and water or prepackaged towelettes
   2. Catheter
   3. Water-soluble lubricant such as K-Y jelly
   4. Storage container for catheter (clean bottle or plastic sandwich bag)
   5. Graduated container to catch and measure urine
B. Procedure for girls
   1. Wash hands well with soap and water.
   2. Wash and rinse between labia from front to back.
   3. Lubricate the tip of a clean catheter.
   4. Insert tip of catheter into the urethra. Continue to advance catheter slowly until urine begins to flow. When the bladder is empty, remove catheter slowly, pausing if urine starts to flow again.
C. Procedure for boys
   1. Wash hands well with soap and water.
   2. Wash and rinse penis starting at the meatus (opening).

(continued)

3. Lubricate the tip of a clean catheter.
4. Hold penis just behind glans (where shaft meets head) and stretch slightly. Insert tip of catheter and advance slowly until urine begins to flow. If slight resistance is encountered, rotate catheter with a twisting motion of the fingers while continuing to slowly advance. If catheter will not advance or if child experiences excess pain, withdraw catheter and consult with parent, physician or supervisor. When urine ceases to flow, slowly withdraw catheter, pausing if urine starts to flow again.

D. Special information for boys and girls
1. Boys may be catheterized while they are lying on a cot or examining table or in their wheelchair.
2. Girls are best catheterized while lying on a firm examining table. A good light is necessary. The outer lips of the labia majora should be spread apart with the finger and drawn upwards. This maneuver exposes the opening of the urethra (small slit-like opening just in front of the vagina.)
3. If no examining table is available and a girl must be catheterized on a cot, place several pads or pillows below her buttocks so the genitalia are easily visible.
4. It is desirable to teach a child self-catheterization, but it is advisable to proceed slowly and not cause undue fears that ultimately could delay self-catheterization. Each child is ready at a different chronological age, depending on his/her cognitive capabilities.
5. For smaller children, the amount of urine recovered will usually be small and may be allowed to run into the diaper unless there are specific orders to measure the amount.
6. When the urine stops flowing, press gently over the bladder area for more complete bladder emptying.

V. WARNING SIGNS

A. There are several signs that are considered to be warning signals of urinary tract infections.
B. Notify parent, supervisor, or school physician if following warning signs are noted:
1. Fever
2. Foul-smelling or cloudy urine
3. Incontinence (constant wetness when fluid intake and interval between catheterization have been correct)
4. Bleeding

(continued)

VI. CATHETER CARE

    A. Red rubber catheter—Wash catheter with soap and water. Rinse well and dry. Store in a dry container (plastic sandwich bag). Replace catheter when it becomes brittle, frays, or loses its shape.

    B. Plastic catheter—Rinse well with tap water both inside and out. Store tube in a straight container (if not, tube will kink or break). Replace tube when it becomes brittle, frayed, or loses its shape.

Pharyngeal and Nasopharyngeal Suctioning

Severely disabled children with an impaired swallowing reflex (usually associated with cerebral palsy) often need suctioning when they choke on their saliva.

Suctioning can be done with a soft rubber bulb or a catheter attached to a suction machine. It is best to have both handy; the bulb to keep near each child for frequent, brief suctioning of small amounts and, less frequently, the machine to clear the deeper nose and throat passages when more thorough suctioning is necessary.

While it is necessary to go through a brief instructional period, this is a technique that can only be mastered by practice following an actual demonstration. For many children it must be performed several times a day, and whoever does it becomes proficient in a short time. As with most procedures, it is best to have a professional school nurse initiate the process in school, instruct the aide or teacher, and observe long enough to insure the procedure is done well.

Colostomy, Ileostomy, Nephrostomy, and Other Ostomy Bags

Changing bags at school is no different from changing them at home or in a doctor's office. The biggest obstacle is getting used to doing this slightly distasteful task in school. After it is done a few times, it becomes as routine as changing a diaper. When the children get old enough they can change their own bags and should be provided with the necessary privacy.

The parents should bring all the necessary paraphernalia: bags, cleansing pads, tape, and whatever else is used at home. The frequency of changes varies completely with the child. Some children have a fresh bag applied at home each morning and never require changing at school. Some require a change of bags at school several times a day, either because the bag fills up or works loose.

Children with an ostomy bag may have no academic deficiencies and may not be in special education. If, for some reason, there is a need for special education or a related service, the child would qualify under the category of "Other Health Impaired."

Tracheostomy

Tracheostomy tubes require special care. They are of two types—a double-walled aluminum tube, and a simpler, single plastic tube. When a child first has a tracheostomy, the double-walled tube is inserted. The outer sleeve is left in place at all times, only being removed by the doctor on special occasions. The inner tube is removed by the parent or nurse whenever it needs to be cleaned. For children who need to retain a tube for months or years, a simpler single plastic tube is used. It can be removed and cleaned whenever necessary because the hole in the throat is permanently open.

It is unusual for a child to be attending school while wearing a tube inserted in the windpipe. Most tracheostomy tubes are put in place for medical emergencies or other temporary conditions, and need to remain in place a few days to a few weeks. However, when children come to school with a tube in place, it is for a chronic condition and may need to remain in place for months or years.

What would happen if the tube were to fall out or be coughed out while the child is at school? Would he choke or die? Fortunately, this would not present an emergency, since the child could continue to breathe through the hole in the throat. There is plenty of time to call the school nurse to replace the tube or to take the child to the doctor. A tracheostomy opening that is relatively new (one to three days old) could close in three to twelve hours (but such a child will not be in school); one that has been in place for several months would take days or weeks to close.

To properly care for a school child with a tracheostomy tube, a professional-quality, portable suction machine is needed. The frequency and type of care needed varies with each child. The doctor should prepare detailed protocols and standing orders if the school nurse is expected to participate in the child's care.

Gastrostomy and Tube Feeding

When a patient cannot be fed by mouth, a short rubber or plastic tube may be inserted directly into the stomach through a surgically created opening in the abdominal wall. Liquid or semiliquid foods are given directly through the gastrostomy tube. The surgeon may leave the tube indwelling or may leave an opening through which the tube is inserted each time the child is fed.

Some children are fed with a tube inserted through the nose, down the back of the throat and into the stomach (a nasogastric tube).

A tube that starts in the mouth is an orogastric tube. Nose and mouth tubes are usually changed every two or three days. If left in place too long, they irritate the lining of the nose and throat.

Whichever type of tube feeding is used, the school nurse should not have to withdraw, insert, or change a tube; this should be done at home by the parent or visiting nurse. The school nurse or health aide will have to give one or two feedings during the school day. For gastrostomy feedings, the school nurse may prefer to insert and withdraw the tube for the noon feeding.

The technique is simple; the liquid food is allowed to slowly run down the tube by gravity, or it can be slowly pushed with a bulb syringe or large (50 cc) hypodermic syringe. After completion of the feeding, enough water should be added to clear the tube. Then the free end of the tube is clamped shut.

If the tube comes out or gets plugged (a rare occurrence), replacing it is never an emergency. There is plenty of time to take the child home to have it replaced. If the school nurse knows how to replace a tube, it is an extra service to the parent, but written permission should be obtained in advance.

OCCUPATIONAL AND PHYSICAL THERAPY
IN THE SCHOOL SYSTEM

Historical Introduction

Occupational therapy (OT) developed in the early 1900s in hospitals for patients with long-term mental and physical illnesses. The word "occupation" meant that the patient would be meaningfully occupied doing physical tasks that would be therapeutically beneficial. The role of the occupational therapist was to develop tasks that patients with chronic mental and physical handicaps could perform and to help the patients perform them. (*American Journal of Occupational Therapy*, March 1987, Robert K. Bing, Ed.D., FAOTA.)

The 1985 guidelines of the American Occupational Therapy Association state, in summary, that a child with a dysfunction in any of the following areas should be referred to OT:

- *Activities of daily living:* self care, home- or schoolwork, play/ leisure, or prevocational/vocational skills
- *Performance components:* neuromuscular, psychological, social, or cognitive development

The 1986 guidelines of the American Physical Therapy Association are more closely oriented to the evaluation and therapy of children with physical and motor disabilities, but they also include assessment and treatment of deficiencies in perceptual-motor development, daily living skills (bathing, dressing, hygiene, etc.), and sensory-motor integration.

It is evident that both OT and PT feel that they should have a large role in the management of *all* children with developmental disabilities.

Historically, the evolution of OT/PT has been in medical institutions. Now, however, a large part of their work is done in schools, so the concepts of a "medical model" emphasizing patient health, and an "educational model" emphasizing student learning have evolved. Because most school districts employ teachers, psychologists, and other educational specialists to meet the individual needs of children with learning and emotional/behavioral problems, OT/PT in schools are best utilized as "motor specialists," primarily serving orthopedically impaired students. The role of the OT/PT, as seen by some school districts, embraces two functions:

- the identification of motor dysfunctions that impede the educational process
- the alleviation of such dysfunction through the use of adaptive equipment and/or therapeutic programming

This is generally seen as the educational model, and the obvious recipients of OT/PT services will be children who have cerebral palsy, muscular dystrophy, or spina bifida, children with orthopedic appliances (braces, splints, crutches, walkers, wheelchairs), and children with other neuromuscular disabilities. Some children with orthopedic or neurologial handicaps do not have any educational handicaps and therefore may not require school-based OT/PT, an obvious example being a child with a well-functioning artificial limb following trauma. (Some would argue that such a child would require school health-related services to provide transportation to and from school. This must be decided by the school evaluation and placement teams.)

Children on the Borderline

There is a sizeable group of children who are categorized as learning disabled, emotionally disturbed, or mentally retarded who are awkward and clumsy, have perceptual-motor disorders, and/or delayed development but do not have any specific musculo-skeletal or neurological abnormality. These children do not need traditional OT/PT services, but they may benefit from adapted classroom or playground activities. It is appropriate for OT/PT to assist teachers in developing group activities to accomplish educational goals such as improved fine or gross motor function or pre-academic skills such as cutting and pasting or using pencils and crayons.

Every year, there should be a group of children who have received maximum benefit from OT/PT. Therefore, apart from appliances and adaptive equipment that require change as the child grows, some children can "graduate" from the need for OT/PT services. The use of a "goals, objectives, and time frame" physician's request form should help school districts select these children.

Role of the School Nurse

Obviously, school nurses do not have the professional expertise to provide OT/PT consultation, evaluation, or therapy. (Also, state nursing practice acts prohibit it.)

However, the relationship between OT/PT, schools, and physicians is still evolving. Since in most schools the school nurse is the overall health service *provider,* she should play a coordinating role between the medical and educational aspects of OT/PT in the following ways:

1. Liaison between the school evaluation team (teacher, counselor, educational diagnostician) and the child's health care provider. Children with any health-related problems who are being evaluated for special education should be evaluated by the school nurse. She should be the person designated to contact the child's physician to ascertain if OT/PT services would be beneficial. Occupational and physical therapists usually feel that they should be the ones to decide whether or not their services would be beneficial to the child. This is not in the best interests of the student; it is not in keeping with the holistic approach, it further fragments patient care, it is more likely to provide continuation of unnecessary services, and it may lead to missed diagnosis of underlying conditions or complications.

2. Coordination of annual physician review of children receiving OT/PT services. The school nurse should see that the child's parent receives the school-designated form and returns it after the doctor has completed it. This is a specialized function and some school nurses may feel it is beyond their expertise. Therefore I recommend that large school districts assign at least one nurse to Special Ed.

Relation to Physician

Traditionally, children's health needs are best met if a pediatrician or family doctor is the overall case manager, referring the child to various medical specialists or paramedical therapists as the need arises. This is often called the "holistic" approach, and it serves children well. Recently, medical care has become more fragmented and more patients are treated by specialists and therapists without any overall coordination. This trend is often seen in large urban school districts. Many economically deprived children have no "medical home base," and those with various developmental disabilities are apt to receive OT/PT services without any physician oversight for long periods of time. This is not only costly, but it poses a danger to children who may receive therapy while postponing a proper diagnosis of the underlying medical condition (for example, a child with early undiagnosed muscular dystrophy receiving perceptual-motor exercises or adapted P.E.).

Therefore, all children with developmental disabilities who are receiving OT/PT services should see a physician at least once a year. Also, a simple note on a standard doctor's prescription blank requesting "OT/PT" should not be acceptable. The school district should develop a form, to be filled out by the doctor, that states the goals and objectives of therapy and the time frames for meeting those goals. If the goals are not met in the stated time period, it can be assumed that therapy did not help and the methods used can be discontinued or altered.

The "Physician's Prescription for Occupational/Physical Therapy," shown on the next page, is a suggested form that school districts can adapt to meet their own needs.

Legal Aspects

The practice of OT/PT is governed by state law. Many states require a physician's prescription for an occupational therapist or physical therapist to evaluate or provide therapy. Some states require the medical prescription only for therapy, not for evaluation. Therapists have developed the concept of "consultation," which may or may not require a physician's prescription. Some therapists feel that if they are "working in the educational model," they may provide services or therapy without any physician oversight at all.

STUDENTS WITH SPECIAL HEALTH NEEDS

The following section is adapted from a position paper entitled "Students With Special Health Needs," by the Health Advisory Committee of the Texas Council of Urban School Districts, May 1987. The paper's lead writers were Marilyn Marcontel, R.N., and Richard Adams, M.D.

More than ever, children with severe disabilities are now attending school. It has become apparent to educators and health professionals that smaller classes, complexity of health services, and different types of equipment are necessary to manage these students properly. A variety of health care professionals is required. A classification system for chronically ill and/or disabled students, based on the amount and type of health care required, will help determine the

**PHYSICIANS' PRESCRIPTION FOR
OCCUPATIONAL/PHYSICAL THERAPY
(circle one or both)**

Student name _____

Date _____

Date of birth _____ School _____

DIAGNOSIS AND BRIEF DESCRIPTION OF DISABILITY:

GOALS OF THERAPY   TIME LIMITS TO ACHIEVE GOALS
(Be as specific as possible.)

SPECIFIC TREATMENT REQUESTED
(Examples: range of motion, daily living skills, active/passive exercises)

SPECIAL PRECAUTIONS AND INSTRUCTIONS

Next appointment with you _____

_____   _____
Printed name of physician   Physician's signature   date

number of health care personnel needed and their necessary level of expertise (R.N., L.V.N., aide).

The following system classifies students according to severity and nature of disability:

1. *Medically complex* students are those with long-standing illnesses that may:

—interfere with education

—require daily or weekly monitoring

—require interpretation to educators

These students may not have observable physical disabilities but, nevertheless, have complex illnesses that often require special attention. Examples are students with asthma, diabetes, or epilepsy.

2. *Medically fragile* students are those with serious long-standing illnesses that usually get worse and are often life threatening. These students may require extensive curriculum adjustments, frequent visits to the doctor, and frequent medication. Examples are students with leukemia, muscular dystrophy, sickle-cell anemia, or AIDS.

NOTE: For these first two categories of students, it is not necessary that a nurse be on the campus every day, but a trained health person should be on call and available within five to fifteen minutes.

3. *Medically intensive* students are those who require a special health procedure one or more times every day or who are subject to cardiac or respiratory arrest or frequent grand mal seizures. Examples of such procedures are naso-gastric tube feedings, tracheostomy care, or catheterization. These children may be profoundly disabled with severe cerebral palsy or be bright little children with spina bifida. Their distinguishing characteristic is their daily requirement for a trained health professional, and at least one school nurse should be on campus every day.

An alternative, simpler classification has been developed by a group of school administrators, school nurses, and doctors working with the Texas Education Agency.

A medically fragile child is one who has a life-threatening condition and requires a skilled professional nurse on campus at all times. Examples are:

1. Students who have exhibited severe episodes of cardiac or respiratory arrest and are in imminent danger of recurrence.

2. Students with severe life-threatening physical deformity, such as extreme hydrocephalus with danger of rupture, or extreme scoliosis or other bone abnormality that may impair the function of a vital organ.

3. Students requiring continuous life support, such as cardiac or apnea monitor, or continuous assisted respiration.

4. Students with severe neurological disorders, such as extreme variations in body temperature, or frequent status epilepticus.

5. Students with tracheostomy or excess pharyngeal secretions that require suctioning more often than every hour.

6. Students with any other medical condition that is permanent and considered by the medical staff to be life threatening without constant medical attention.

The chronically ill child with special health needs is usually cared for at home by his/her parents. The parent is trained by the doctor or nurse to carry out whatever procedures are necessary, for example, tracheostomy suction or catheterization. When the child is well enough to go to school, the usual assumption is that the school nurse will do whatever procedures must be done during the school day. However, because each procedure takes only a few minutes and there is rarely a nurse at all schools every day, health aides may be trained to do it.

This may seem like a practical solution, but it is legally risky. The school district may have to prove in court that a health aide is sufficiently skilled to perform these tasks. A professional school nurse, therefore, should try to perform all procedures of this nature if at all possible.

Specialized equipment, such as catheters, diapers, ostomy bags, tracheostomy tubes, and suction machines may be required. Some states have ruled that medically related equipment must be furnished by parents; in other states, school districts will furnish some and ask parents to provide other equipment. Usually a school district will buy a suction machine or a small oxygen tank if the equipment is to remain at the school and be used for more than one child. The parents are expected to furnish catheters, suction tips, and diapers—supplies that are disposable or used only for a single child.

If specific district policy or state law does not apply, the school district should address each case individually, taking into account parental ability and severity of handicap, and always act for the maximum benefit to the child.

Least Restrictive Environment

One of the major dilemmas a school district must face involves school placement of a child with a severe or profound disability. Federal law requires the child be placed in the least restrictive setting consistent with his/her educational and health needs. This was never intended to mean that *all* disabled children be placed in mainstream schools. Nevertheless, some parents and educators are interpreting it this way. An individual child's health needs may require daily skilled nursing care. The child's neighborhood school may have a nurse only one or two days a week, whereas a special school usually has a full-time nurse who is skilled at performing specialized procedures. Also, the special school has needed medical equipment.

Some disabled children, particularly those with severe mental retardation, function better socially and educationally in a special school. Also, their health needs can be better met there. It is often a mistake for educators to place these children in a mainstream school merely to meet a supposed federal guideline.

Because each child's disability is unique, individual decisions must be made in every case. Particular difficulties arise when the physical disability is severe but there is no cognitive deficit. With such cases, everyone involved should have one or a series of informal meetings (with no one taking notes) and agree on a reasonable course of action. This should occur prior to the formal meetings required by federal and state guidelines. It should include, at a minimum, the parents, the school nurse, the principal, and the teacher. Any of the parties should be allowed to bring a colleague or advocate. It is important that school personnel avoid an adversarial position, because legal procedures are costly. If the case goes to a court of law, sympathy for the disabled child places the district at a disadvantage. If requests are at all reasonable, the district is usually better off acceding to parental requests.

SPINA BIFIDA

Nature of the Condition

Spina bifida, or *myelomeningocele,* is a failure of the vertebral bones (spinal column) to fuse, leaving the enclosed spinal cord unprotected. While this may occur anywhere from the neck to the tail bone, the most common location is the lower part of the spine just above the buttocks. In addition, the skin and spinal cord do not develop properly, and a pouch varying from the size of a walnut to a grapefruit often is present where the bones fail to fuse. (See Figure 20–1). This pouch contains all of the nerves of the spinal cord that are supposed to go to the lower pelvis and legs. In a typical case, the child has no control over bowel or bladder and both legs are paralyzed.

Hydrocephalus (water on the brain) is often associated with spina bifida. This can be prevented or controlled with proper treatment.

In children with a large pouch, the skin is often very thin and may leak spinal fluid. This can also be surgically corrected.

Spina bifida occulta (hidden spina bifida) is a condition in which the failure of fusion of the lower spinal vertebrae is slight and there is no outpouching of the skin, and there are little or no spinal nerve abnormalities. In most cases there are no bladder or bowel symptoms or leg involvement.

Unless there are obvious abnormalities of the brain, and usually there are not, children with spina bifida are emotionally and intellectu-

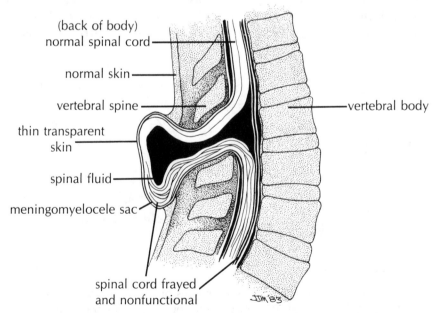

Figure 20–1. Myelomeningocele. (The spinal fluid completely surrounds the spinal cord and is immediately below the skin of the sac. The skin consists only of a thin membrane, which often ruptures spontaneously.)

ally normal. With proper treatment and training, they should be able to attend school. Indeed, there are now many children with properly treated spina bifida attending school in regular classes with normal children. They have equal potential for learning.

Spina bifida associations exist in many large cities. Parents of these children, like parents of all handicapped children, have special needs, and organizations of this nature are very helpful.

Upper extremity problems are common. Since the defect is in the lower back, there is a tendency to assume that the arms are normal. Many children with spina bifida have mild weakness, poor fine motor control, poor awareness of the position of their arms and hands, and poor eye-hand coordination. The upper extremity problems may be overlooked, so awareness of them is important.

Diagnosis and Symptoms

Because of the size of the pouch, the diagnosis is usually made at birth. There are mild cases in which the bones almost fuse and the visible pouch is very small. In these cases, the nerve damage may be slight, and the resulting bowel or bladder or leg paralysis problem may also be slight. (See Figure 20–2.) In cases of this nature, urinary or

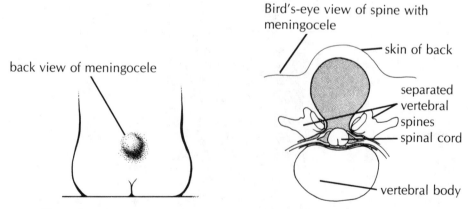

Figure 20–2. Meningocele. The meninges or sac that contains the spinal fluid is pouched out between the separated vertebral spines, but the spinal cord itself is normal. The skin is of near normal thickness. The person has little to no paralysis and may have normal bladder and bowel functions.

fecal incontinence or clumsiness in walking may be noticeable, and the child should be referred to a physician for evaluation.

Spina bifida occulta often causes no symptoms whatsoever. Symptoms such as enuresis, bowel problems, or sensory or motor lower extremity problems may be caused by a variety of other conditions and must be referred to a physician for diagnosis and initiation of treatment. About 20 percent of all children who, for unrelated reasons, receive X-rays of the lower spine will show a tiny failure of the closure of the vertebral bones. Some of these children will also have enuresis or encopresis (bowel soiling). Many years ago spina bifida occulta was thought to be a cause of bed wetting. Currently, most authorities feel there is no cause-and-effect relationship between this incidental X-ray finding and a urinary or fecal problem. In questionable cases, investigation by a neurologist or urologist must be made.

Treatment

Primary treatment of spina bifida is surgical. Since this condition is so complicated and has medical, social, and educational aspects, the entire treatment team must include a pediatrician, a neurosurgeon, a urologist, an orthopedist, a social worker, an occupational therapist, and a physical therapist, as well as the school nurse.

Total treatment consists of the following major procedures, which will already have been done by the time the child starts school:

1. Repair of the skin defect in the lower back
2. Shunt-type procedures in the brain to prevent or arrest hydrocephalus
3. Orthopedic procedures to the legs to enable the child to walk with braces and crutches at an appropriate time
4. Urological evaluation to determine the best method of bladder management

However, even after school attendance begins, medical consultation and some surgical procedures may be necessary throughout the patient's lifetime.

School Relevance and Role of the School Nurse

A typical spina bifida child of school age will already have had the surgery listed above. In addition, many children require diapers and diaper changes for fecal and/or urinary incontinence.

The school nurse may be asked to monitor and consult with the physician in the following areas:

Skin of the Lower Back

Usually very little care is required. Occasionally, however, the scar may become infected, become dry and itchy, or develop crusts. Treatment is to remove crusts gently, apply antibiotic ointment if necessary for infection, cleanse with antibacterial soap, or occasionally apply softening lotions.

Bowel Care

Because of lack of muscular control of the anal opening, fecal soiling is common. Changes of diapers or other appropriate clothing must be kept at school. Privacy and due regard for the child's sensitivities are essential.

Bladder Care

Because of lack of nerve supply to the bladder, the urge to urinate does not exist. Therefore, the bladder fills until it can hold no more, and eventually urine dribbles out of the urethra and keeps the clothes or diaper constantly wet. Since the bladder never empties, the remaining urine and bladder wall often become infected. Modern management requires that the bladder be emptied periodically to prevent infection and subsequent kidney damage. Some older children have learned to empty their bladders by lower abdominal pressure, but most urologists feel that intermittent catheterization every four to six hours is the preferred method. Many school nurses now perform this procedure. It is usually performed once a day at school at about noon. Close contact and consultation must be maintained between school nurse, parent, and physician. School nurses will require a little extra inservice training if they have not performed this procedure for a long time, but the technique is quite simple and can be learned (or relearned) in a short time. Many urologists teach young children self-catheterization. The age at which children can do this varies depending on individual ability, and is usually between seven and ten years. In these cases, the school nurse should work closely with the principal to provide the space and privacy and to make other necessary arrangements.

Care of the Legs, Braces, and Crutches

The school nurse should be aware of possible pressure sores from braces. Sometimes, extra padding may be necessary. Occasionally, notification to the parents or physician for an adjustment will be necessary. Observation of the child while walking will reveal whether the crutches are of proper length and whether the child is using them properly. Occupational and physical therapy are usually necessary.

Observation of Head Size

A child with spina bifida should be brought into the clinic each month or two to have head circumference recorded on the health card. Though there may be an intracranial shunt, its valves occasionally malfunction. Therefore, any unusual head growth—more than ½ inch in six months—should be reported to the parent and/or physician.

Class Placement and Learning Problems

Most spina bifida children can be mainstreamed into regular classes. Many, however, have specific learning problems and poor fine motor control because of subtle cerebral defects (also called perceptual problems). Therefore, psychometric evaluations may be helpful in preparing an individual educational plan (IEP).

Special Problems at Adolescence

As would be expected, depression frequently occurs. Girls worry about childbearing and boys worry about potency. Normal experiences with children of the opposite sex are lacking. Most adolescents need to know more about their condition; their parents have been told, but they haven't. The school nurse and school counselor can be most helpful. A peer group rap session with other handicapped and normal children may give an adolescent an opportunity to express his or her anxieties. The local spina bifida parents' association is the best resource.

MENTAL RETARDATION

Nature of the Condition

There are two major categories of mental retardation—high-level and low-level. The diagnostic nomenclature varies from state to state. Also, medical designations are sometimes different from educational designations.

High-Level

In the recent past, many school systems designated children with an IQ between 70 and 90 as "educable mentally retarded." Some school systems still do. The educational diagnosis is made from the scores on the IQ test and ability to learn basic academic material— reading, writing, spelling, and arithmetic.

Health specialists and some psychologists are reluctant to make a diagnosis of mental retardation at this high level, because observation of this type of child over long periods of time has shown that about two-thirds of them become normal adults: they marry, work, raise children, and function as well as adults who were not so categorized when they were young school children.

Low-Level

Children with measured IQ scores of about 50 to 70 are sometimes called "trainable mentally retarded" or mentally defective.

The American Association for Mental Deficiency has developed an official classification system that is based on the degree of mental and physical retardation. The higher-level children in this category have an IQ of about 50 to 70; the best example is a child with mongolism, or Down's Syndrome. The lowest level in this category is the child who is physically and mentally retarded, completely bedridden, must be tube fed, and gives no indication of any awareness of surroundings. This type of child acquires no self-help skills and requires complete custodial care.

Diagnosis and Symptoms

High-Level

There are no overt symptoms or signs. Academic performance and IQ testing are the only diagnostic clues. On casual observation the child looks, acts, speaks, and understands about as well as other children. Physical ability is usually normal or close to normal. However, first- to third-grade school work is performed very poorly, if at all. Brain functions most seriously affected are memory, spatial relationships, and sequencing ability—those functions most likely to affect learning of basic academic material.

The medical background is usually normal. Walking and talking usually begin at a normal age, as do tricycle riding and toilet training. Socialization with peers at ages three, four, and five is usually normal.

Most parents of children in this category see their children as normal in all respects until they start school. That is why it is so difficult for a parent to accept a diagnosis of mental retardation in a child of this nature. Indeed, public pressure against this diagnosis has finally led many school systems to discard the category from their classifications for special children. Also, the score on an IQ test has been criticized as being much too restrictive as a sole measure of intelligence. In many ways, the IQ test is simply another achievement test rather than a test of anything innate. Provided all other factors are equal, a child who grows up in a nurturing, reading family will perform better (score higher) on an IQ test than that same child would if he or she grew up in a nonnurturing, nonreading environment.

Low-Level

There are many signs and symptoms. The medical or developmental history reveals delays in many functions, motor as well as cognitive. Crawling and walking occur late. Language comprehension is poor from a very early age, and spoken language may never develop at all.

The incidence of convulsive seizures is much higher than in the normal population.

The facial appearance is often abnormal. In many cases the features are broad and thick, the mouth often remains open, and the brow is narrow. The ears may be low-set or unusually shaped. In medical jargon, these abnormalities are called *stigmata*.

Many identified syndromes are associated with chromosomal or metabolic abnormalities plus mental retardation. These syndromes usually have two or three names, one after the individual who first described it and another that is descriptive of the disorder. Dr. John L. H. Down first described the condition, characterized in part by a peculiar eye configuration, hence the term *mongolism*. Other characteristics are short, stubby fingers and a peculiar crease in the palm of the hand. In the past twenty years it has been discovered that the twenty-first chromosome has three parts instead of the normal two, so now the disease is sometimes referred to as trisomy-21. There are more than 100 well-defined syndromes associated with low-level mental retardation. More are discovered and described each year. (See Bergsma's *Birth Defects Compendium*.)

Treatment

High-Level

As a group, these children are physically and emotionally normal. They have no increased susceptibility to disease and need no special care. They can participate in all school activity.

Low-Level

A great deal of nursing care is necessary in this group of children. The amount depends on the degree of retardation.

Children who are high on the scale of low-level retardation can usually be trained to feed themselves and handle their own toilet needs; however, they usually need help until they are at least six years of age.

Because of poor personal hygiene, the incidence of impetigo is higher.

The incidence of impacted ear wax is much higher in mentally retarded children. It is rarely serious enough to interfere with hearing, but as the wax continues to collect, it should be irrigated and washed out periodically. The child can be referred to a physician, or the school nurse, if properly trained, can perform this function. If school nurses are to perform this procedure, they must first learn to use an otoscope and demonstrate proficiency under supervision. The wax must first be softened with an appropriate solution and then irrigated with a gentle stream of water. There are several ear-wax–softening agents available. Two commonly used are Cerumenex™ and Debrox™. Cerumenex™ is stronger, slightly irritating to the skin, and requires a prescription. It works better but should not be given to parents to use at home. It should be dropped into the ear, allowed to remain for thirty to sixty minutes, and then washed out. Debrox™ is completely nonirritating and does not require a prescription. The parent may use it at home for three to five days before the ear irrigation. In either case, the procedure may have to be repeated one or two times. If the child complains of pain, the procedure should be stopped and repeated two or three days later if a sizable amount of wax remains.

Mentally retarded children who have seizures tend to have them more frequently and more severely than nonretarded epileptic children. Some fall and hit their heads so often they must wear protective helmets at all times. The treatment is the same as described in the section on epilepsy. The incidence of *status epilepticus*, however, is significantly higher, so this group of children must be watched more closely.

BIBLIOGRAPHICAL
REFERENCES

Accardo, P. J., and A. J. Capute. *The Pediatrician and the Developmentally Delayed Child.* Baltimore: University Park Press, 1979.

Ayers, A. J. "Improving Academic Scores through Sensory Integration." *Journal of Learning Disabilities* 5:339, 1972.

Barlos, D. "Sexually Transmitted Disease." *The Facts.* New York: Oxford University Press, 1979.

Behrman, R. E., and Vaughn, V. C. *Nelson Textbook of Pediatrics;* 13th ed. Philadelphia: W. B. Saunders Co., 1987.

Bergsma, D. *Birth Defects Compendium;* 2nd edition. White Plains, N.Y.: Alan R. Liss, Inc., 1979.

Cott, A. "Megavitamins. The Orthomolecular Approach to Behavioral Disorders and Learning Disability." *Academic Therapy* 7:245–58, 1972.

Cruikshank, W. M. *Learning Disabilities in Home, School, and Community.* Syracuse: Syracuse University Press, 1977.

De Angelis, Catherine. *Pediatric Primary Care.* Boston: Little, Brown and Company, 1979.

Diagnostic and Statistical Manual of Mental Disorders. Washington: American Psychiatric Association, 1987.

Doman, R. J., et al. "Children with Severe Brain Injury; Neurologic Organization in Terms of Mobility." *JAMA* 174:257–62, 1966.

Faas, Larry A. *The Emotionally Disturbed Child.* Springfield: C. C. Thomas, 1975.

Feigin, R. D., and J. D. Cherry. *Textbook of Pediatric Infectious Diseases;* 2nd edition. Philadelphia: W. B. Saunders Company, 1987.

Feingold, B. *Why Your Child Is Hyperactive.* New York: Random House, 1975.

Friedman, S. B., and Hoekelman, R. A. *Behavioral Pediatrics.* New York: McGraw Hill, 1980.

Gabel, S., Gerald, D., Butnik, S. *Understanding Psychological Testing in Children.* Plenum Medical Book Co., 1987.

Golden, G. S. *Textbook of Pediatric Neurology.* Plenum Medical Book Co., 1987.

Golden, G. S. "Nonstandard Therapies in Developmental Disabilities." *American Journal of Disease of Children* 134:487–91, 1980.

Gubbay, S. S. *The Clumsy Child.* Philadelphia: W. B. Saunders Company, 1975.

Helfer. R. E. *Childhood Comes First.* Lansing: R. E. Helfer, 1978.

Hervett, Frank M. "Strategies of Special Education." *Pediatric Clinics of North America* 20, no. 3, 1973.

Kempe, C. H., and R. E. Helfer. *Helping the Battered Child and His Family.* Philadelphia: Lippincott, 1972.

Kephart, N. C. *The Slow Learner in the Classroom.* Columbus: Charles Merrill, 1960.

King, A., and C. Nicol. *Venereal Disease,* 3rd edition. Baltimore: Williams and Wilkins, 1975.

Kinsbourne, M., and P. J. Caplan. *Children's Learning and Attention Problems.* Boston: Little, Brown and Company, 1979.

Kovacs, M., and A. T. Beck. "An Empirical Clinical Approach toward a Definition of Childhood Depression." In J. G. Schulerbrandt and A. Raskin (eds.), *Depression in Children, Diagnosis, Treatment, and Conceptual Models.* New York: Rowan Press, 1977.

Lazar, P. "Hair Analysis: What Does It Tell Us?" *JAMA* 229:1908–9, 1974.

Lefkowits, M. M., and N. Burton. *Psychological Bulletin* 85, no. 4, 716–26.

Lerner, J. *Children with Learning Disabilities,* 2nd edition. Boston: Houghton Mifflin, 1976.

Levine, M. D., and J. P. Shankoff. *A Pediatric Approach to Learning Disabilities.* New York: John Wiley and Sons, 1980.

Levine, M. D. *Developmental Variation and Learning Disorders.* Educators Publishing Service, 1987.

Lewis, K., and Thomson, H. *Manual of School Health.* Addison Wesley, 1987.

Morbidity and Mortality Weekly Report, Rabies Prevention, U.S. Dept. of Health and Human Services, June 13, 1980.

Murdek, G. C. "The Abused Child and the School System," *American Journal of Public Health,* 60:105–9, 1970.

Paluzny, Maria J. *Autism: A Practical Guide for Parents and Professionals.* Syracuse: Syracuse University Press, 1979.

Parcel, Guy. *Teaching My Parents about Asthma.* Galveston: University of Texas Medical Branch, 1976.

Philpott, W. H., et al. "Allergic States in Children with Learning Problems." Read before the Ninth International Congress of ACLD. Atlantic City, N.J., February 1972.

Rutter, M. "Diagnosis and Definition of Childhood Autism." *Journal of Autism and Childhood Schizophrenia* 8:139–61, June 1978.

Safer, D. J., and R. P. Allen. *Hyperactive Children.* Baltimore: University Park Press, 1976.

Silver, L. B. "Acceptable and Controversial Approaches to Treating Learning Disability." *Pediatrics* 55:406–15, 1975.

Vaughan, D., and T. Asbury. *General Ophthalmology,* 8th edition. Los Altos, CA: Lange Medical Publications, 1977.

Weston, H. C. *Sight, Light, and Efficiency.* London: H. K. Lewis and Company, 1949.

Zanga, Joseph R. *Manual of Pediatric Emergencies.* Churchill Livingstone, 1987.

INDEX